Health into Mathematics

Longman Group UK Limited,
Longman House, Burnt Mill, Harlow,
Essex CM20 2JE, England
and Associated Companies throughout the world

First published 1991

Set in 10/12pt Plantin

Printed in Malaysia
by Percetakan Jiwabaru Sdn. Bhd.,
Ipoh, Perak Darul Ridzuan

ISBN 0 582 05839 2

Contents

Preface

A CHALLENGE TO THE TEACHER

This book does not provide a formal set of exercises. Regard it as a set of suggestions, of sample ideas from which you can select activities which will work in your class. You can decide when and where to slip the health lesson into the mathematics you teach.

If children are taught subjects in tight little boxes they will think of them as separate and unconnected. The ideas in this book are intended to stimulate you to think of more activities that cross the artificial barrier between mathematics and health education.

A CHALLENGE TO THE CURRICULUM WRITER

If you looked at a primary mathematics syllabus from any country in the world you would find it hard to tell from which country it comes. Most syllabi are very similar and take little account of the particular problems faced by primary school leavers in different countries.

Here is a challenge to curriculum writers to develop mathematics materials infused with the health education needed in your country. This is an opportunity for curriculum development to avoid being a reflection of that in another country and to be a response to the needs and priorities of your own educational system.

A CHALLENGE TO THE EXAM WRITER

The primary school leaving examination plays a dominating and sometimes tyrannical role in determining what teachers actually teach. The exam writer has immense power but with that power goes responsibility: responsibility for improving the mathematical education provided in schools. One positive contribution an exam writer can make is to include questions which integrate health and mathematics and by so doing set an example of the way in which a student's understanding of the relevance of mathematics to other aspects of life may be deepened.

Acknowledgements

The Health Across the Curriculum series

In 1987, Hugh Hawes of Child-to-Child and Beverley Young of the British Council first discussed the possibility of a Health Across the Curriculum project. Building on the experience of Child-to-Child, the idea was to develop a series of books for teachers, helping them to understand how they could link health education with other areas of the curriculum. Several African countries expressed their willingness to participate in and support the project, each concentrating on a particular curriculum area.

Funded by the British Council and Child-to-Child, workshops to develop the idea and plan the writing were held as follows:

Country	*Title of Book*	*Date*
Kenya	Health into Mathematics	1987
Zimbabwe	Health into Science	1988
Uganda	Health into Social Studies	1989
Botswana/Lesotho	Health into Language	1990 (planned)

This book, Health into Mathematics, is the first of the series. It was written by William Gibbs and Peter Mutunga. The initial workshop at which the book was planned took place in Kenya in September 1987 and was attended by the authors, John Webb, Freda Nturibi, Murray Macrae, Joseph Chumo, Bryan Wilson, and Norman Nzioka under the guidance of Michael Kinunda. These, and many others in Kenya and the UK provided practical details, creative ideas and sound advice, all of which was invaluable in the creation of this book.

All the photographs in this book were supplied by William Gibbs.

The Child-to-Child Trust is based at the Institute of Education and the Institute of Child Health at London University. It produces valuable activity sheets and story books for children on all the health themes examined in this book. A particularly useful resource book for health education in schools, which uses the child-to-child approach, is Young and Durston's *Primary Health Education* (Longman, 1987). All these child-to-child materials as well as other low cost books and studies in health education, are available from Teaching Aids at Low Cost, P.O. Box 49, St. Albans, Herts, England, AL1 4AX.

How to use this book

This is a book of activities for use in primary schools. It is not a textbook to be followed page by page, but rather a source of ideas. There are two main ways in which we suggest you use the book:

1 **To bring examples from health education into your mathematics teaching.**

In Part A of the book you will find three chapters with the headings 'Statistics and Health', 'Teaching about Health through Ratios', and 'Teaching Health through Percentage'. If you are teaching one of these maths topics then look in the relevant chapter for activities which can also be used to develop a health message. Use the contents list at the front of the book to find the topics that interest you or turn to the **health into mathematics chart** at the back of the book for a summary of all the health activities relevant to the maths topic you are teaching. Beside each activity you will see the words 'Lower', 'Middle' or 'Upper'. This is the level in the primary school at which this activity will be most suitable.

2 **To bring mathematics into health education.**

In Part B of the book you will find chapters with headings such as 'Nutrition and Breast Feeding' and 'Body and Growth Monitoring'. These chapters will tell you more about the important health messages that children can learn. They also suggest many mathematical activities that will help the children learn about health and mathematics at the same time.

Adapting the activities to suit your needs.

When you have found an activity you would like to use, you may have to adapt it so that it suits your children and your classroom. Many of the activities in this book are based on the Kenyan environment so there are references to Kenyan names and Kenyan statistics. This shows that it is possible to make mathematics relate to the health concerns of a particular society. Because of this you may want to adapt the names and data in some activities so they refer to your country and are then as relevant as possible to your students.

Introduction

The network of primary schools spread throughout a country provides a powerful channel through which health education can flow to every community. In the past, health education has been limited to a few periods a week on the primary school timetable; sometimes it is little more than a cleanliness inspection at the start of each day. By contrast, mathematics is a high-status subject with a prominent position on the timetable.

This book is part of the *Health Across the Curriculum* project which aims to find and develop links between health teaching and the major subjects taught in primary schools.

In particular this book looks at ways of slipping health information and knowledge into mathematics lessons.

This will have two powerful results. The amount of health education will be increased and the learning of mathematics will be enriched by being related to the life and experience of the child.

THE HEALTH PRIORITIES

The World Health Organization has called for 'Health for all by the year 2000'. This is not a dream but is based on the power of primary health care to improve dramatically the state of the world's health.

Primary health care does not mean more doctors and hospitals. It means involving everyone, teachers, families, communities and children in a campaign of increased responsibility for their own health. It concentrates on attacking those barriers to good health which can be demolished by increased knowledge and endeavour in the home, in the village and in the school.

The primary school teacher has an important role to play. Not only is the teacher in contact with the children in the classroom, but through them with their families and the whole community. It is vital that primary school teachers are aware of the priorities of health care and of the influence they can have in improving the health of their class, their school and of the larger community.

Here then are the six important topics in health education.

Body and growth monitoring

A sensitive and effective way to make sure children are growing properly is to measure their weight at regular intervals. Health clinics keep a record of each child's development on a growth chart.

The increasing use and understanding of growth charts can have a dramatic effect on the pinpointing of children at risk from disease and malnutrition.

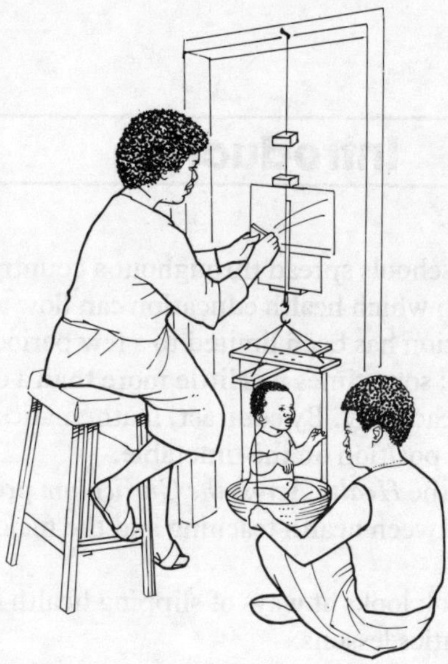

The child is weighed regularly and the weight recorded on a growth chart

Nutrition and breast feeding

Children who do not eat the right balance of food do not grow to full height or weight, nor is full mental and intellectual growth possible.

A one-year-old child is about $\frac{1}{6}$ of the weight of an adult

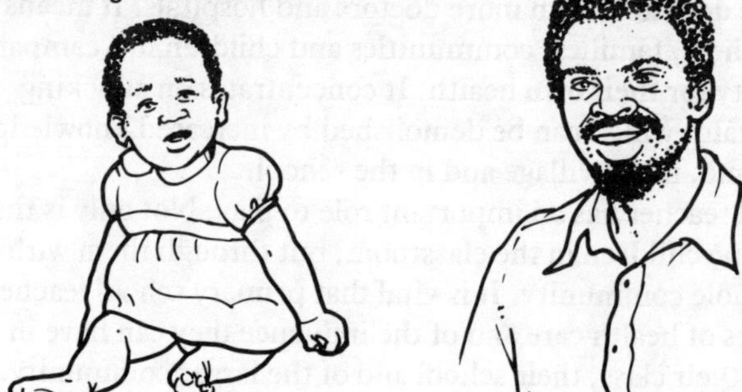

but the child needs to eat about $\frac{1}{2}$ the amount an adult eats

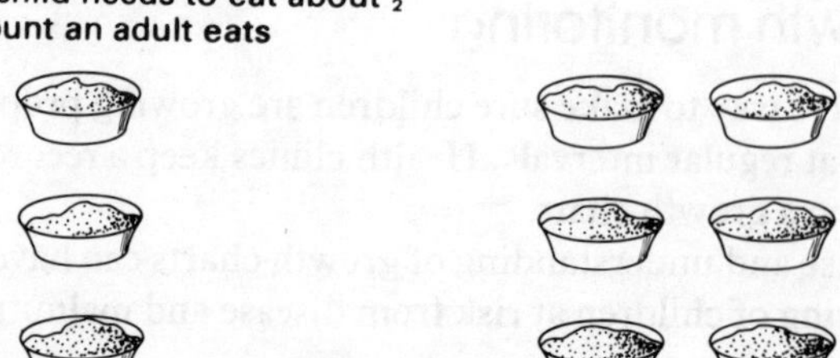

Population

The attempts to raise the quality of life and provide a reasonably healthy life for all are hindered by the high rate of population growth.

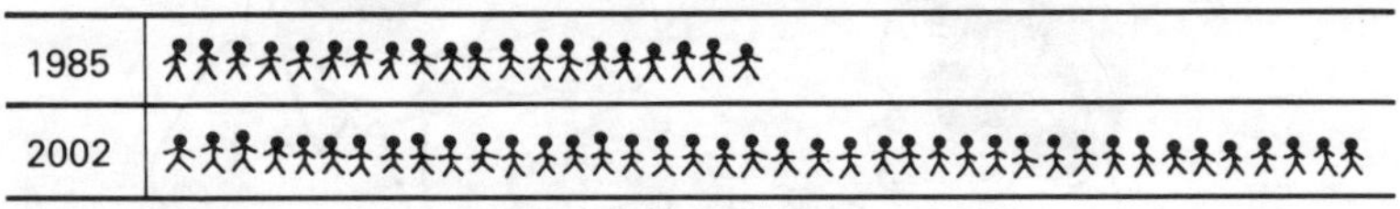

In 17 years the population of Kenya will double

= 1 million people

Infectious diseases and immunization

Deadly illnesses can be abolished by immunization.

The increased effectiveness of immunization campaigns depends on the active cooperation of the community.

Only 26% of children in the developing world are vaccinated against measles

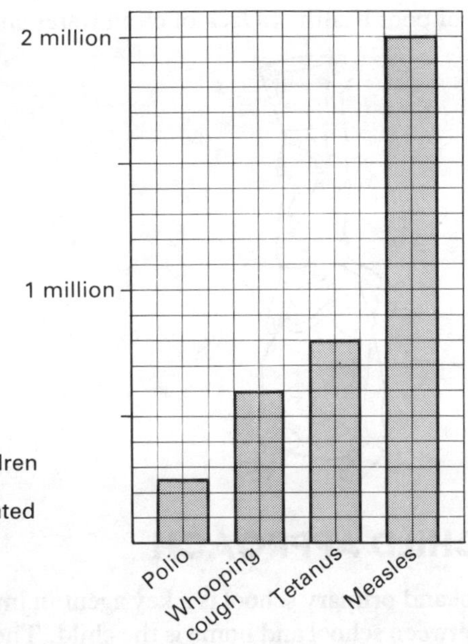

Deaths every year in the world from diseases which can be prevented by vaccine

Treating diarrhoea: sugar–salt solution

The sugar–salt solution is a mixture of sugar, salt and water. It helps to prevent dehydration which results from diarrhoea and is a simple medicine that children can learn to make.

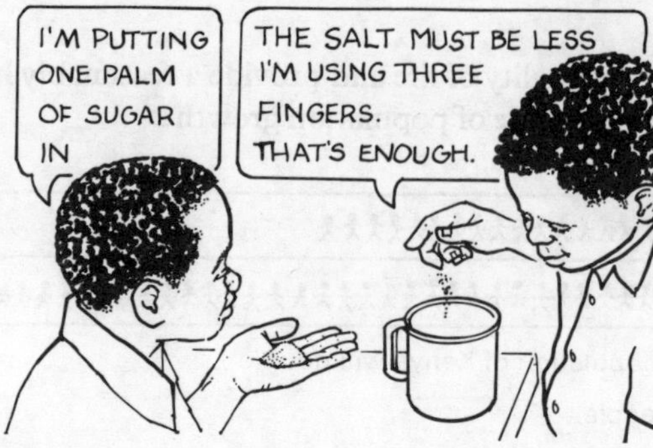
I'M PUTTING ONE PALM OF SUGAR IN
THE SALT MUST BE LESS I'M USING THREE FINGERS. THAT'S ENOUGH.

The sugar–salt solution can prevent 20% of the 14 million deaths a year among the world's under-fives

Water and sanitation

One of the major causes of poor health is a lack of clean water and sanitation.

Average distance to water:
dry season 1.2 km
wet season 0.7 km

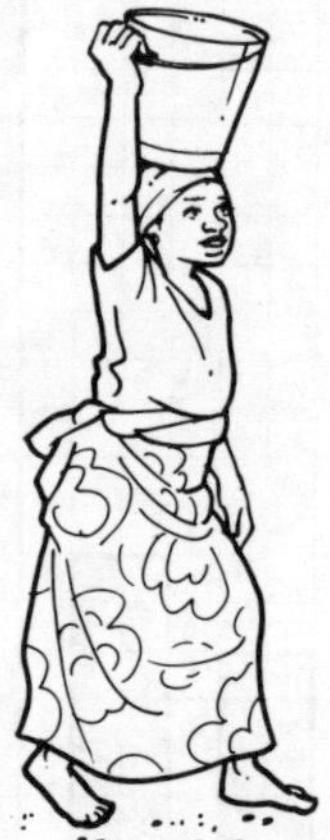

THE CHILD-TO-CHILD APPROACH

The teacher in pre-school and primary school is a key agent in improving health education but the link between school and home is the child. The child-to-child approach is based on the belief that the school-age child can play a vital role in health education in both the home and the community.

School children can

- take health information from school to home,
- bring information about health in the home to school,
- share information with children of the same age at home and at school,
- improve the health care of younger brothers and sisters.

In many countries older children spend a lot of time helping to look after and care for their younger brothers and sisters. The child-to-child approach is to use the child as a major agent of health care.

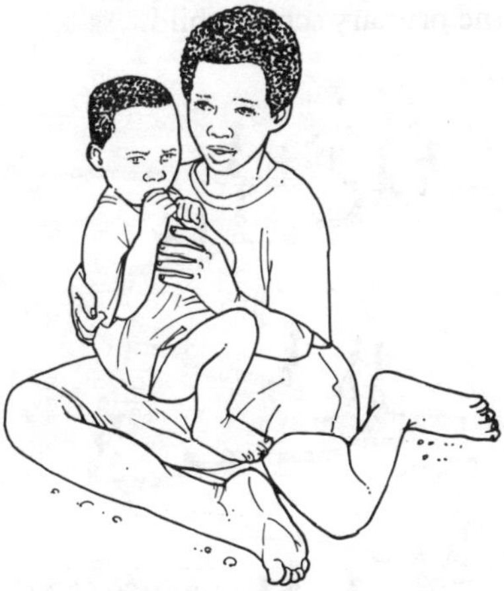

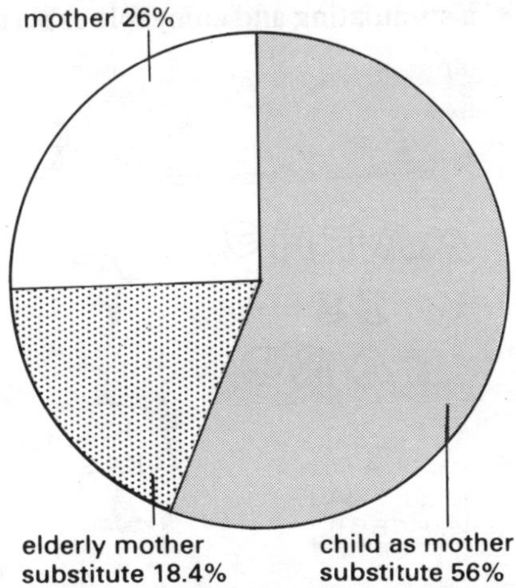

Who provides child care?

Many of the activities included in this book involve children in collecting information about their families, their households and their communities. Other activities suggest ways in which school children can monitor the growth and well-being of their younger brothers and sisters, and yet others suggest ways in which older children can act as 'little teachers', helping younger ones to develop mental skills.

All these activities are marked with the child-to-child logo.

The child-to-child logo

WHY TEACH HEALTH IN MATHEMATICS LESSONS?

There are conflicting views about the role of mathematics in the primary school. There are those who see mathematics as essentially

- a hard subject at which most children will fail,
- an isolated abstract convention,
- an abstract course which successfully selects the able from the less able,
- an unpleasant subject which inevitably the majority of children will not wish to study.

In contrast there are those who see primary mathematics as

- of value to all,
- related to other aspects of life,
- understandable through concrete and practical experiences,
- a stimulating and enjoyable experience for the primary school child.

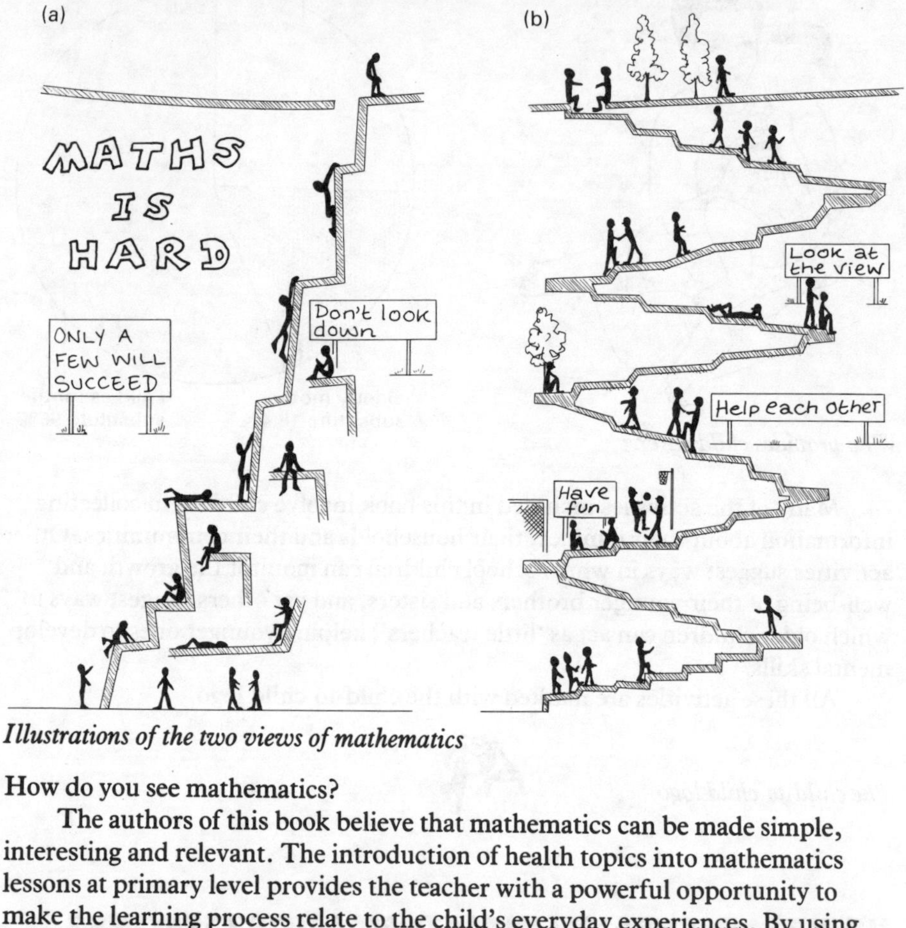

Illustrations of the two views of mathematics

How do you see mathematics?

The authors of this book believe that mathematics can be made simple, interesting and relevant. The introduction of health topics into mathematics lessons at primary level provides the teacher with a powerful opportunity to make the learning process relate to the child's everyday experiences. By using examples and problems that are concerned with the growth of children and the health of the community the teacher can make classroom mathematics more real, alive and easier to understand.

How can health and mathematics be integrated?

Look at the diagrams that illustrated the health priorities.
Can the ideas shown be used in a health lesson?
Could they be used in a maths lesson?
Which topics in maths does each link with?

INTRODUCING THE HEALTH INTO MATHEMATICS CHART

When we started collecting ideas for this book we drew up a chart with the health priorities down the left-hand side and the main mathematical components of the primary syllabus along the top.

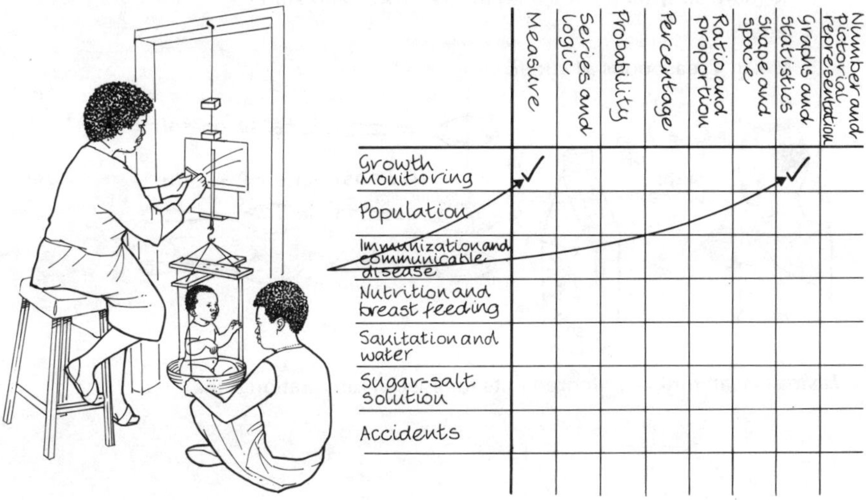

First version of health into mathematics chart

Each box on the chart represented the intersection of a health topic and a maths topic. We then tried to think of activities that fitted the boxes. For example, the weighing of children and the recording of the weight on a chart is growth monitoring but it also involves measurement and the use of graphs. So we put ticks in two boxes on the chart as shown above.

Here are some more health activities. Can you decide which boxes on the chart to tick for each one?

(a)

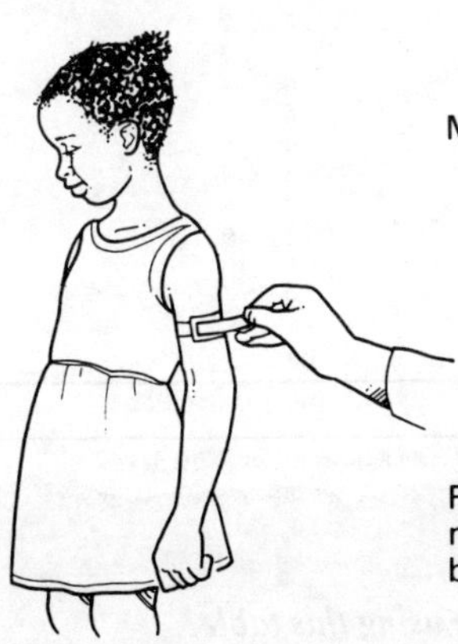

Measuring round the arm

From the first to the fifth birthday a measuring strip has provided a simple but satisfactory assessment of nutrition.

(b) Special rehydration drink

1 Find a family-sized soft fizzy drink bottle (750) ml) and wash it out.
2 Fill the bottle with clean drinking water.
3 Mix in $\frac{1}{2}$ teaspoon of salt.
4 Taste the drink. It should taste like tears. If it is more salty than tears then throw it away and start again.
5 Mix in 4 teaspoons of sugar.

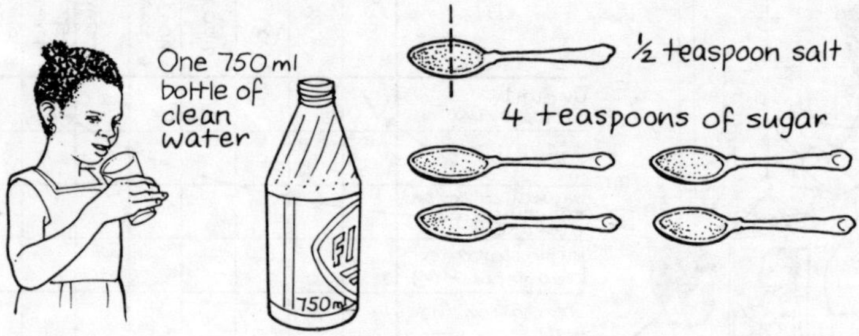

Taste special drink Ingredients for special rehydration drink

(c)

The ten most common infant and child diseases, 1978

Disease	Infants (< 1 year)	Ranking	Children (1–4 years)	Ranking
Pneumonia	26	1	21	2
Enteritis and other diarrhoeal diseases	21	2	10	3
Measles	10	3	23	1
Malaria	6	4	8	4
Acute respiratory infections	5	5	4	6
Bronchitis, emphysema and asthma	4	6	5	5
Tetanus	3	7	–	–
Symptoms and ill defined conditions	2	8	2	10
Anaemias	2	9	3	7
Meningitis	1	10	–	–
Burns	–	–	3	8
Avitaminoses	–	–	3	9
Others others	20		18	
Total all cases:	100		100	

Source: R.O.K., Ministry of Health, Health Information Bulletin, Vol: 4, No. 4, 1982.

What mathematics can you demonstrate using this table?

Our chart looked similar to the figure below. In some columns there are no ticks. Each row in the chart was ticked, showing that each major health topic included a mathematical element.

	Measure	Series and Logic	Probability	Percentage	Ratio and proportion	Shape and space	Graphs and statistics	Number and pictorial representation
Growth Monitoring	✓				✓		✓	
Population		✓		✓	✓		✓	✓
Immunization and communicable disease			✓	✓	✓		✓	✓
Nutrition and breast feeding	✓			✓	✓		✓	✓
Sanitation and water	✓			✓			✓	✓
Sugar-salt solution	✓			✓	✓		✓	
Accidents			✓				✓	

The final health into mathematics chart contains fewer columns but gives details of relevant activities in each box. All the activities suggested in this book for a particular maths topic can be found by looking down the columns. All the activities for a health topic can be found by looking along the rows.

The health into mathematics chart may be found at the back of the book.

PART A

Health into mathematics

1 Statistics and health

Statistics in the primary school is concerned with

- collecting information in class, around the school and at home,
- displaying information, for example, by making graphs, drawing bar charts or pie charts,
- asking and answering questions about the information.

Often statistics becomes a dull and arid topic in school. The information collected has no meaning for the child, the display has no purpose and there is no reason for the questions asked.

One way to give the statistics taught in primary school meaning, purpose and relevance is to base it on the health issues and problems within the community. Asking the right questions and drawing the relevant graphs can heighten children's awareness of health priorities. Seeing problems more clearly is often the first step towards finding a solution.

Teaching health through statistics allows children to

- find out more about the health and health needs of themselves, their friends, their families, and their communities,
- learn the mathematical skills of statistics in a practical and relevant way.

TEACHING STATISTICS

Children start by collecting and displaying information about themselves. They can make simple graphs using themselves or regular objects.

Here is an activity which combines statistics and population.

- Activity 1 — Lower
- **Position in the family**

Get the children to sort themselves into groups, all the first-born in one group, all the second-born in another, and so on.

Ask the children to arrange themselves so that it is easy to compare the size of each group.

The children in each group stand in line. To make the spacing equal the children stand so that they can just touch the shoulders of the child in front. The children have made a graph (see Plate 1).

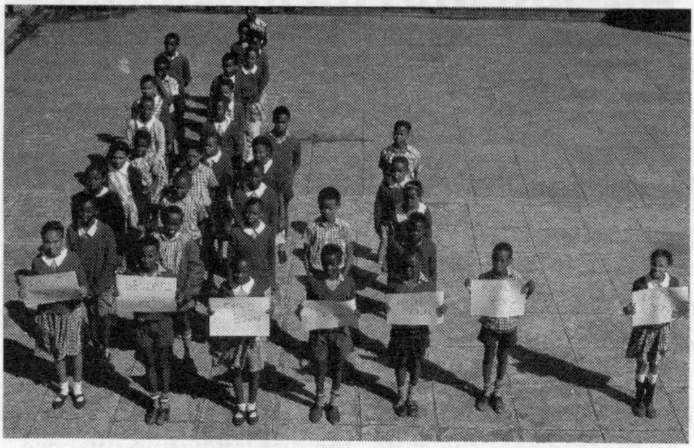

Plate 1 Children's graph of family position

After using themselves to make the graph, the children can make a similar picture using exercise books on the floor or matchboxes built into towers.

Another way to display information simply is in a pictogram. The next activity shows a simple way for the class to create a pictogram.

• Activity 2 — Lower

• Last illness

Each child has a piece of paper of the same size. On the paper the children each draw a picture of themselves. Discuss with the children the illness they had last. Make a list of the illnesses and then build up a pictogram with the children's pictures. Each child can pin or place their pictures alongside the illness they had last.

The children can make a pictogram of the same information on squared paper. In figure 1-1 each drawing of a stick person stands for one child.

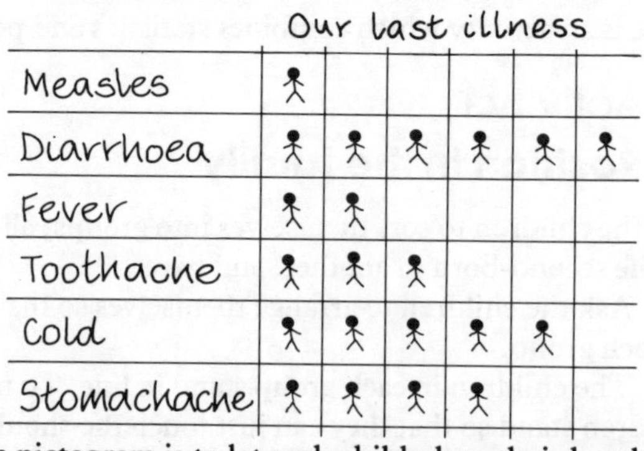

1-1 Children's pictogram using squared paper

Another way of making a pictogram is to let each child place their hand on the blackboard in line with their last illness. Then the child draws around his hand. A pictogram of handprints will be created.

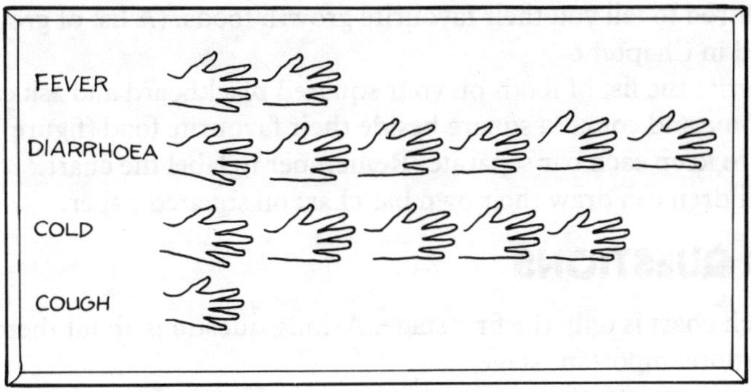

1-2 Hand-print pictogram

For more activities on illness see Chapter 7.

COLOURING SQUARES TO MAKE A BAR CHART

Once the children have made pictograms on squared paper it is but a little step forward to make a bar chart. To make a class bar chart it is a great help to have a squared blackboard. For hints on how to make one see the Appendix.

- Activity 3 **Middle**
- **Our favourite growth foods**

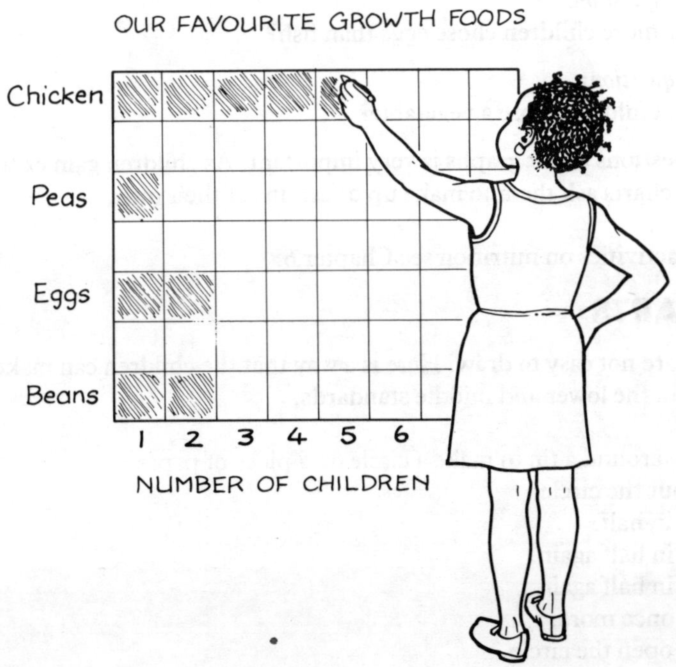

1-3

Ask the children to tell you their favourite growth foods. (A list of growth foods can be found in Chapter 6.)

Then write the list of foods on your squared blackboard and ask each child in turn to come and colour a square beside their favourite food (figure 1–3). Remember to keep each bar separate. Remember to label the chart.

The children can draw their own bar chart on squared paper.

ASKING QUESTIONS

Drawing each chart is only the first stage. Asking questions about them is the second and more important stage.

There are a variety of questions you can ask. Here are some examples:

'How many?' questions
How many children chose chicken?
How many chose beans?

'Which?' questions
Which food was chosen by 4 people?
Which food was chosen by 2 people?

'Comparison' questions
Did more children choose beans or eggs?
Which food was chosen by most children?

'Difference' questions
How many more children chose eggs than fish?

'Addition' questions
How many children chose a vegetable?

Asking questions about graphs is very important. As children gain experience of looking at charts ask them to make up questions of their own.

For more activities on nutrition see Chapter 6.

PIE CHARTS

Pie charts are not easy to draw. Here is a way that the children can make simple pie charts in the lower and middle standards.

(i) Draw around a tin to make a circle on a piece of paper.
(ii) Cut out the circle.
(iii) Fold in half.
(iv) Fold in half again.
(v) Fold in half again.
(vi) Fold once more.
(vii) Now open the circle.

The creases on the paper divide the circle into 16 equal parts. Here is an example of an activity that will use this circle to make a pie chart.

• Activity 4 — Middle

• Our favourite energy foods

Ask the children to list five energy foods. (A list of energy foods can be found in Chapter 6.)

Each child asks 16 others in the class to choose their favourite. The results of the survey can then be recorded by the children in a tally chart (see figure 1-4).

(a)

Energy Foods

Rice	✓	✓	✓				
Potatoes	✓	✓	✓	✓			
Bananas	✓	✓	✓				
Nuts	✓	✓	✓				
Bread	✓	✓	✓				

After collecting the information the children can colour their circle to show the results of their survey.

(b)

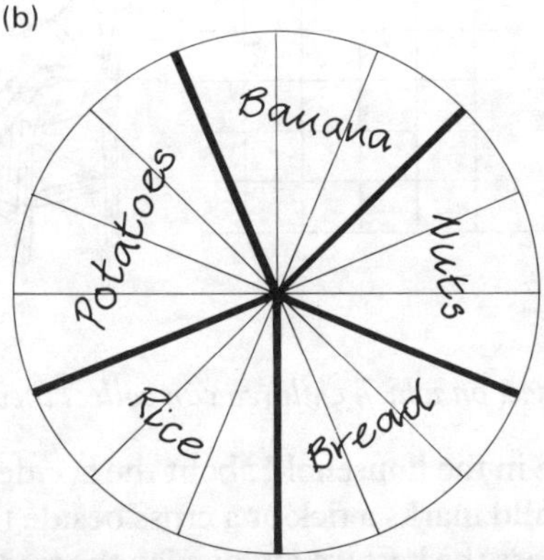

1-4 Favourite 'Go' foods: (a) Children's tally chart (b) Children's pie chart

STATISTICS AND ACCIDENTS

Here are examples of a series of activities which help children to learn about statistics and about health.

• Activity 5 — Lower/middle
• My last accident

Ask each child to remember the last accident that happened to them.

Make up a list of the accidents and use it to build up a bar chart on the blackboard. Each child then colours in one square.

The children can then make their own record of the chart, make up questions and answer them.

Discuss the results found with the class, the cause of common accidents and ways of preventing them.

• Activity 6 — Middle
• Accidents in the household

After making simple charts from information collected inside the class, the children can make up a survey to be carried out in their homes.

The questions to be asked need to be decided in class and a simple way of recording information prepared. Figure 1-5 shows an example of the record they could make.

Accidents in my home

Name					
Broken bone					
Cut needing stitches					
Severe burn					
Snake bite					
Scorpion sting					
Poisoning					
Road accident					

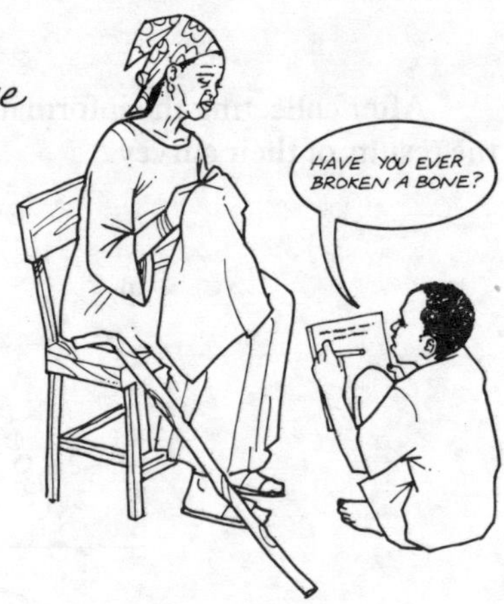

1-5 Example of record sheet on which children can collect their own data at home

The child asks everyone in the household about the accidents they have had. Below their name the child marks a tick or a cross beside the accident.

Discuss with the class the best way to display the findings of the survey. Each child might make their own bar chart or the class might divide into groups and each group draw a bar chart showing their results.

The question of scale will naturally arise from this activity. The children will need to decide whether 1 square stands for 1, 2 or 4 or more accidents.

- The children can make up questions on their charts for other groups to answer.
- The children can compare the charts made by each group and discuss which accidents can be prevented and how.

• Activity 7 — Middle

• How do cuts happen?

Here is another example of a home survey that children can carry out. The children make up a list of the objects that are likely to cause cuts. They can ask each member of their household if they have ever been cut by each of the objects.

How cuts happen

Name	Liban	Naima		
Tin	✗	✗		
Knife	✓	✓		
Axe	✗	✗		
Pin	✗	✗		
Glass	✓	✗		
Thorn	✗	✓		
Razor blade	✗	✗		

1-6 Example of record sheet for home survey

Figure 1-6 is an example of the record sheet they might prepare. The results can be made into charts and discussed.

• Activity 8 — Middle

• Road accidents

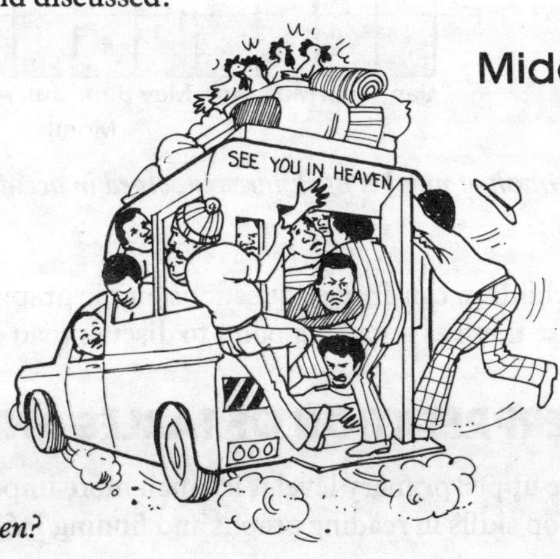

1-7 What do you think might happen?

Once the children have collected their own information and shown it in the form of a chart it is much easier for them to read and interpret graphs and charts made by others.

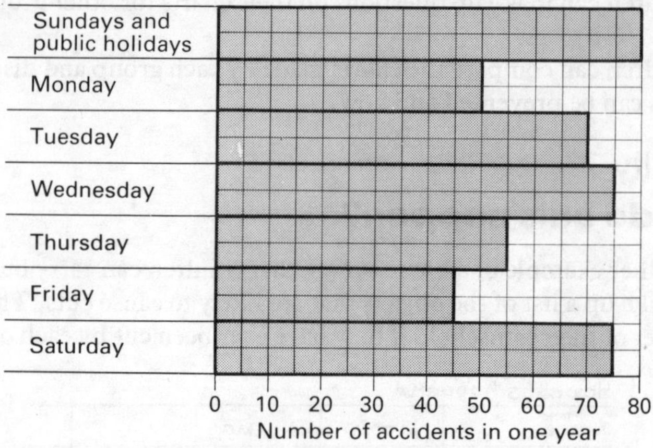

1-8 Graph of days on which accidents happen in Nairobi

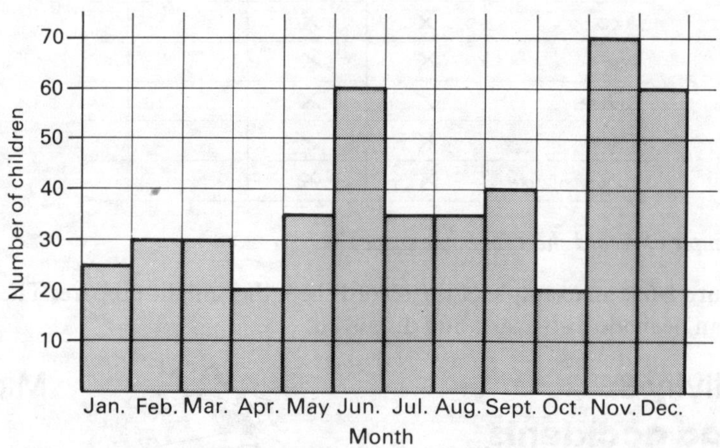

1-9 Graph of number of children involved in accidents in Nairobi each month

The children can answer questions on the graphs in figures 1-8 and 1-9 and you can use them as a starting point to discuss road safety.

INTERPRETATION OF TABLES AND GRAPHS

At the upper primary level it is much more important that children should develop skills in reading graphs and finding information from tables than drawing up their own. Here are examples of various types of information displayed in different ways. Each provides an exercise in developing skills in reading and understanding numerical and graphical information. Each has a health application.

These examples may stimulate you to find similar tables and graphs that you can use to deepen the mathematical skills and health knowledge of your pupils.

• Activity 9 Lower

• When to take medicines

Here is a simple method that is used by health workers to remind people who cannot read how much medicine to take.

The day is divided into 4 parts (see figure 1-10(a)).

(a)

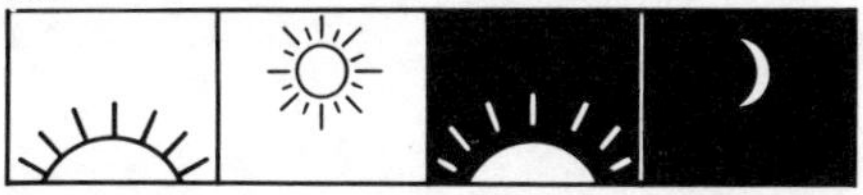

This picture below means 1 tablet, 4 times a day.

(b)

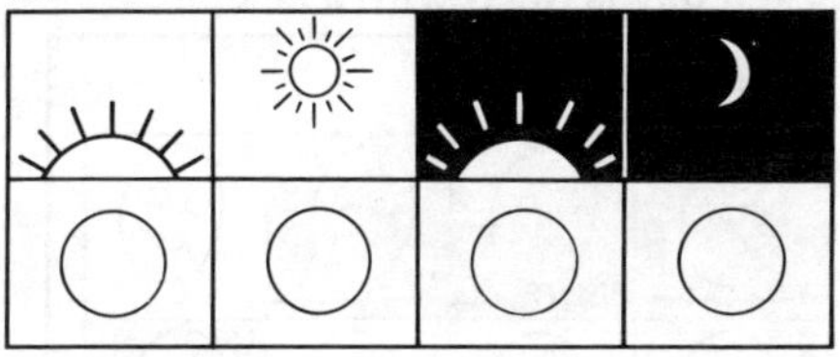

This picture below means ½ tablet, 2 times a day.

(c)

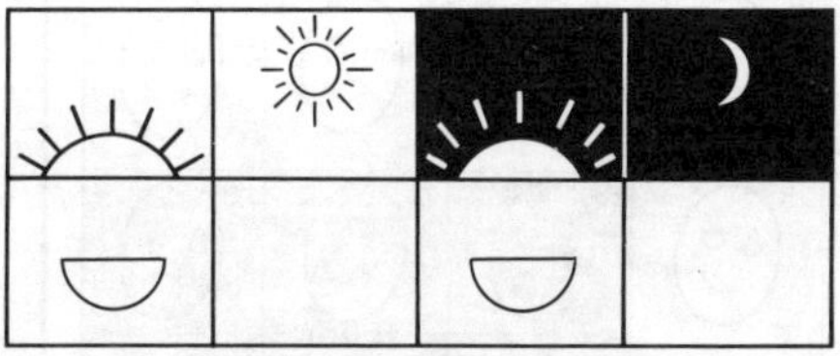

The children can work out what the pictures mean in the rest of figure 1-10.

(d)

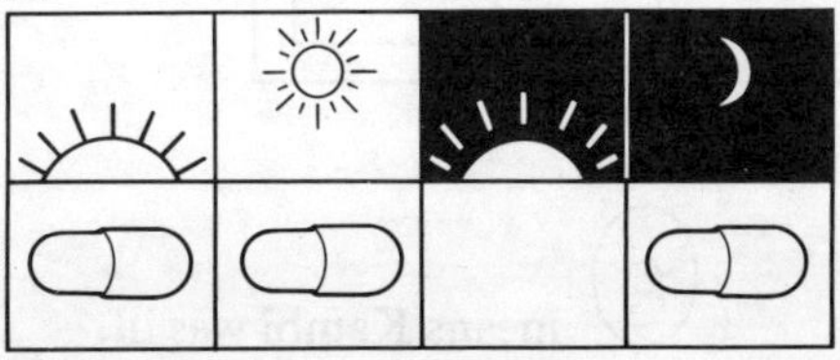

(e)

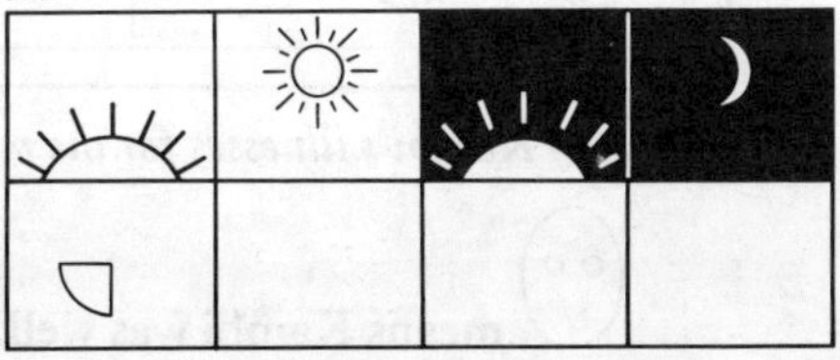

(f)

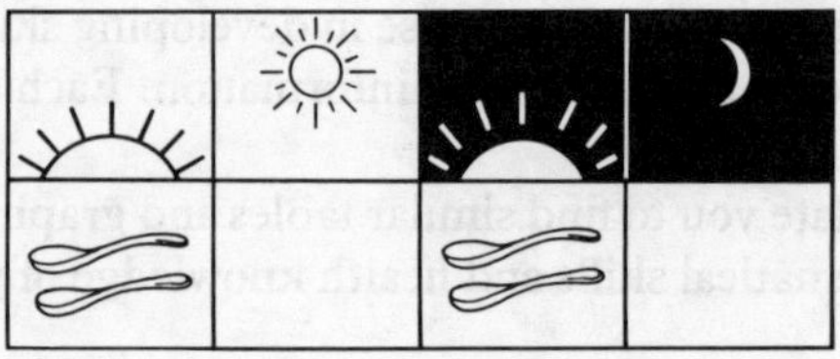

1-10 Simple pictures giving instructions for taking tablets

The children can draw their own pictures to show other instructions, for example,

- 1 tablet, 2 times a day,
- 1 capsule, once a day,
- $\frac{1}{4}$ tablet, 4 times a day,
- 3 teaspoons, 3 times a day.

• Activity 10 — Lower

• Illness chart

Figure 1-11 is a sickness chart for the month of June for a child called Kambi. The chart is like a calendar; each day is filled with a face.

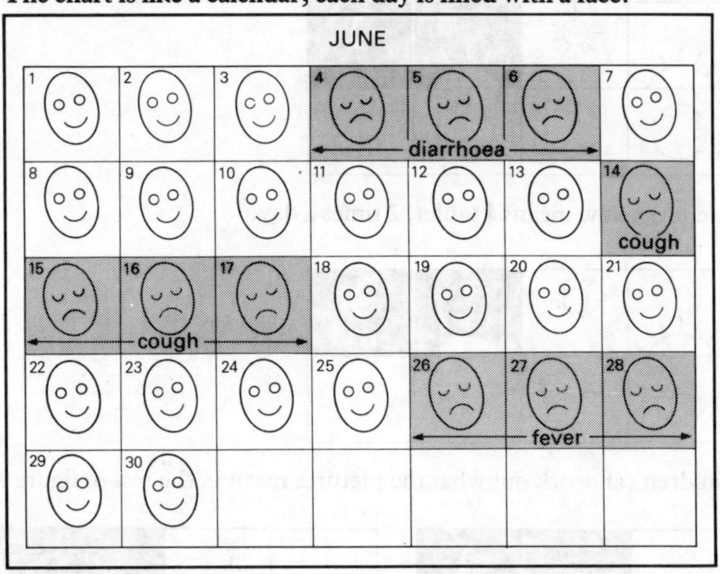

1-11 Chart of Kambi's illnesses for the month of June

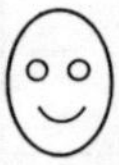 means Kambi was well.  means Kambi was ill.

The children can answer questions on the chart, for example,

- How many days did Kambi have diarrhoea?
- Which illness lasted four days?
- How many days was Kambi sick during the month?

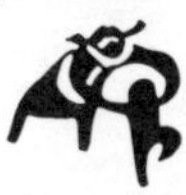

The children can make up a chart like this for a baby brother or sister. They can draw in a face for each day. At the end of the month discuss the charts with the children. Remind them that when young children are ill, they do not eat well. They need to make up this lost food on other days.

For more activities on illness see Chapter 7.

• Activity 11 Upper

• Infant death rate

Many children die in their first year. The number dying is recorded in every country in the world. The percentage of babies who die in their first year is called the *infant death rate*.

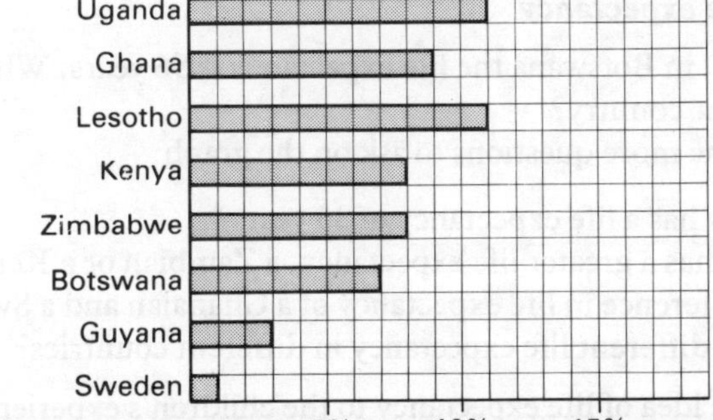

1-12 Chart showing ***infant death rate***

For example, in Zambia the rate is 8% (see figure 1-12). This means that 8 out of every 100 children born will die in the first year of life.

Here are some more questions to ask on the chart:

- What is the infant death rate in your country?
- Which country has a rate of 16%?
- Which country has the highest rate?
- Which country has the lowest?
- Why do you think there is so great a difference?

• Activity 12 Upper

• Life expectancy

The average number of years that people live is called *life expectancy*. The life expectancy is not the same in all countries, as you can see from the graph in figure 1–13.

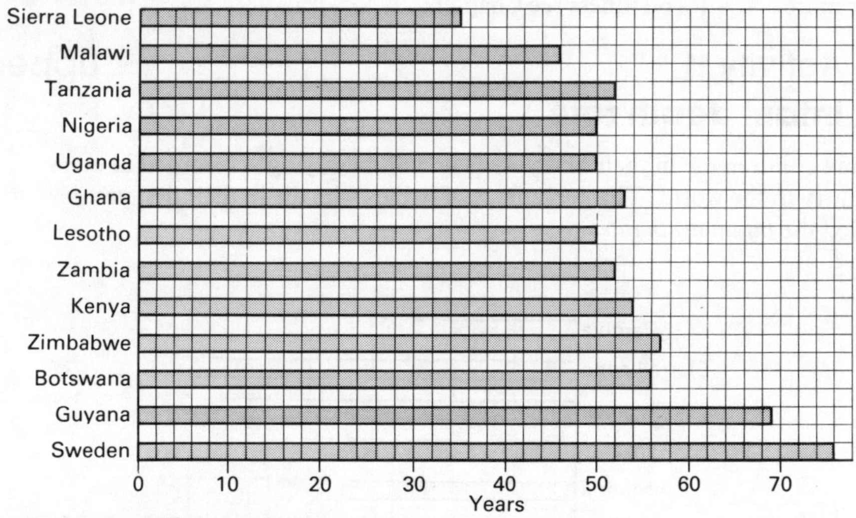

*1-13 Graph of **life expectancy***

For example, in Botswana the life expectancy is 56 years. What is the life expectancy in your country?

Here are some more questions to ask on the graph:

- Which country has a life expectancy of 35 years?
- Which person has a greater life expectancy, a Zambian or a Kenyan?
- What is the difference in life expectancy of a Ghanaian and a Swede?
- Why is there a different life expectancy in different countries?

To relate the idea of life expectancy to the children's experience, ask how many of the class have all four grandparents living, how many have three living, two living, one living, or none. Find out the age of their oldest living relative.

• Activity 13 Upper

• Population pictogram

To make a classroom pictogram of population the children can use the paper folding method to create people chains (see page 82). Each cut-out figure stands for 1 million people. The children can make people chains to show the populations of countries in Africa (see figure 1-14).

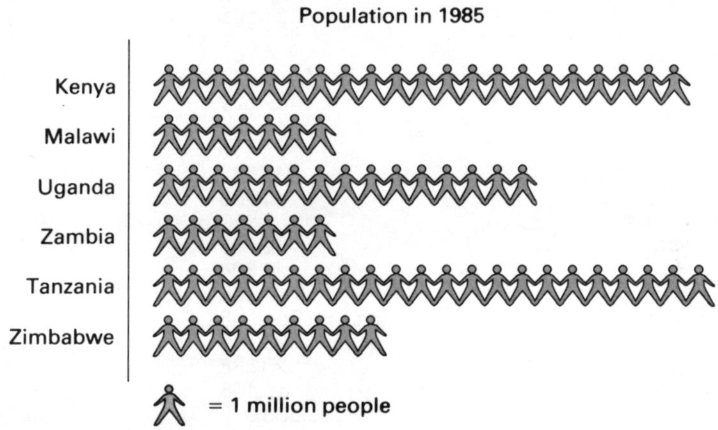

1-14 Population in 1985 shown by people chains

For more activities on population see Chapter 5.

• Activity 14 Upper

• Population statistics

Each country publishes the results of its surveys on population in statistical bulletins.

Such data provide an opportunity for a good deal of simple numerical problem solving using large numbers. They can also provide very good practice in rounding figures to the nearest hundred or thousand or million.

Here are some examples of possible questions on Table 1-1:

- How many more Kikuyu females are there than males?
- What is the total number of Turkana?
- Does any group have more males than females?
- What is the total male population to the nearest million?

The children will be interested in their own group. Ask them to compare it in size with other groups to find where it ranks in order of size. Ask them to make up mathematical sentences of their own using the data in the table.

For more activities on population see Chapter 5.

Table 1–1 Kenyan population census 1979
Population by sex, tribe, race and nationality

Tribe or nationality	Male	Female
Kenyans		
Kikuyu	1 582 145	1 620 676
Embu	89 471	90 929
Meru	416 800	423 704
Mbere	29 242	32 483
Kamba	852 360	873 209
Tharaka	4 763	4 919
Luhya	1 048 914	1 070 794
Kisii	469 629	474 458
Kuria	46 388	42 781
Mijikenda	357 116	375 714
Pokomo	19 835	19 906
Taita	74 068	79 051
Taveta	3 850	3 826
Swahili/Shirazi	2 903	2 743
Bajun	18 304	18 667
Boni/Sanye	2 108	2 062
Luo	966 548	989 297
Kalenjin	820 749	831 494
Masai	120 838	120 557
Samburu	36 168	37 457
Turkana	106 009	101 240
Teso	66 192	66 295
Nderobo	3 698	3 502
Njemps	3 668	3 878
Rendille	10 940	10 854
Boran	35 306	33 588
Gabbra	15 467	15 086
Sakuye	926	898
Orma	16 134	15 993
Gosha	917	935
Hawiyah	811	793
Ogaden	13 584	12 058
Ajuran	11 309	10 697
Gurreh	41 901	41 182
Degodia	49 227	43 808
Somali (so stated)	83 119	72 575
Basuba	29 889	29 779
El Molo	277	261
Asian	17 402	15 152
European	2 200	2 245
Arab	9 486	9 375
Other Kenyans	29 711	27 607
Total Kenyans	**7 510 372**	**7 632 528**
Non-Kenyans		
Africans	39 744	32 074
Asians	23 755	22 291
Europeans	17 409	18 047
Arabs	10 562	9 723
Others	5 102	5 111
Total Non-Kenyans	**96 572**	**87 246**
Not stated	169	174

• Activity 15 Upper

• Comparing graphs about common diseases

Comparing two charts or two sets of information can often be a valuable exercise. The two charts in figure 1-15 show the four most common diseases of children in Kenya. The children are divided into two groups: those under 1 year old and those between 1 and 4 years old.

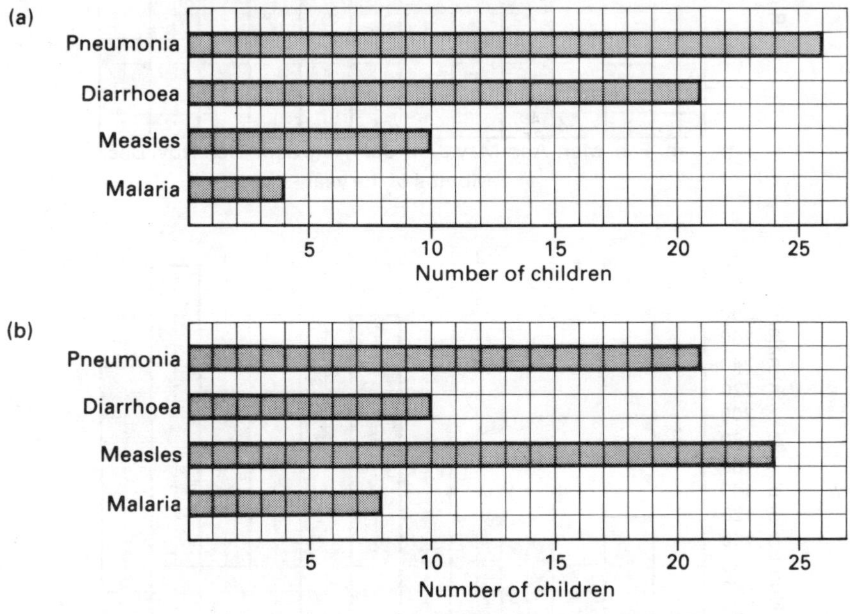

1-15 (a) Children under one year old treated by village clinic (b) Children between one and four years old treated by village clinic.

The children can compare the two charts and make simple statements. For example: The most common disease for children under 1 year old is pneumonia. For children between 1 and 4 years old, it is measles. (Pneumonia is an acute infection of the lungs, often coming after other breathing illnesses.)

For more activities on diseases see Chapter 7.

• Activity 16 Upper

• Relating graphs about malaria and rainfall

Putting information in graphs often helps us to see the connection between two things and to deduce the cause of an effect.

The children can answer simple questions on each of the charts in figure 1-16.

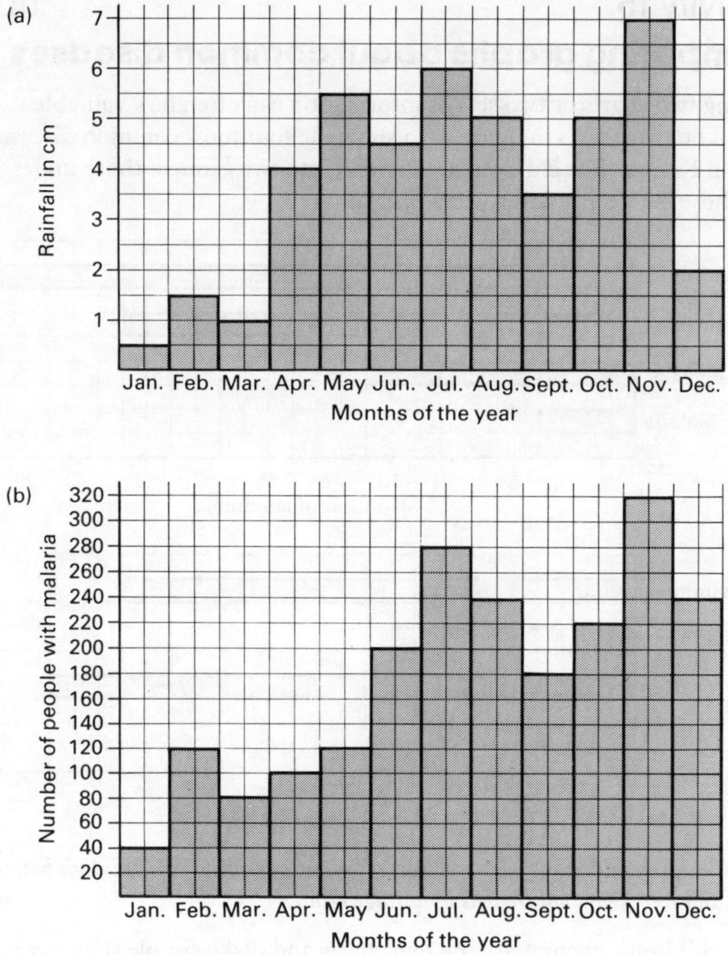

1-16 (a) Rainfall in Karamoja (b) Malaria in Karamoja

- How much rain fell in May?
- How many cases of malaria were there in June?

Then children can study the two charts and look for connections between them. The guiding questions are:

- Which months have the highest rainfall?
- When is malaria most common?

Children can deduce for themselves that an increase in the number of people with malaria is linked to increased rainfall. Ask them to explain why.

Now the children can try to predict what happens in other countries with a different pattern of rainfall. When will most cases of malaria be found in Nigeria? (Figure 1-17)

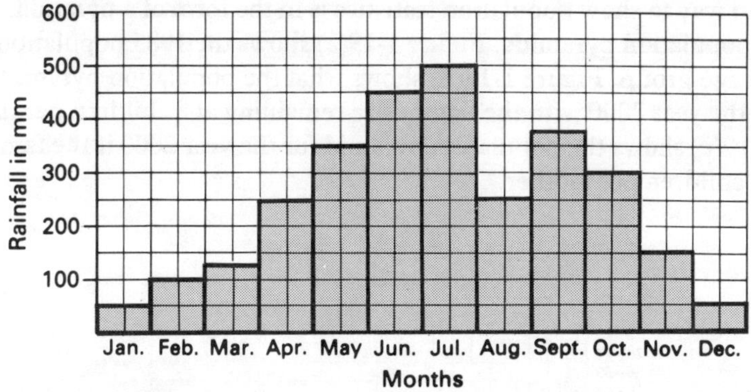

1-17 Rainfall in Nigeria

For more activities on diseases see Chapter 7.

• Activity 17 Upper

• Pie charts of how work is shared

The pie charts in figure 1-18 show how some of the daily household jobs are shared between men and women in Kenya.

The children can make statements based on each pie chart. They can also make comparisons between the charts.

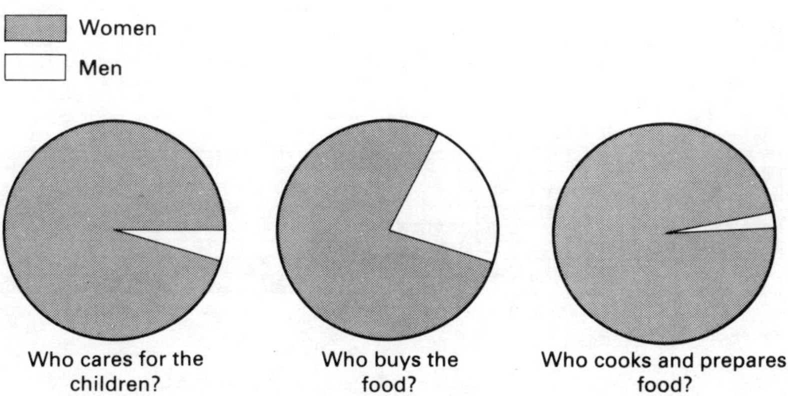

1-18

Health message: Do not neglect the girls in your class. They will play a very important part in the health of the next generation.

• Activity 18 Upper

• Population pyramids

A common way to show population statistics is in the form of a pyramid. Here are three population pyramids. Figure 1-19(a) shows the 1985 population of Kenya by age-group. Figure 1-19(b) shows what the population pyramid might be like in the year 2000 with the family size remaining at 8 children per mother. Figure 1-19(c) shows the population pyramid for the year 2000 if the family size became 4 children per mother.

(a)

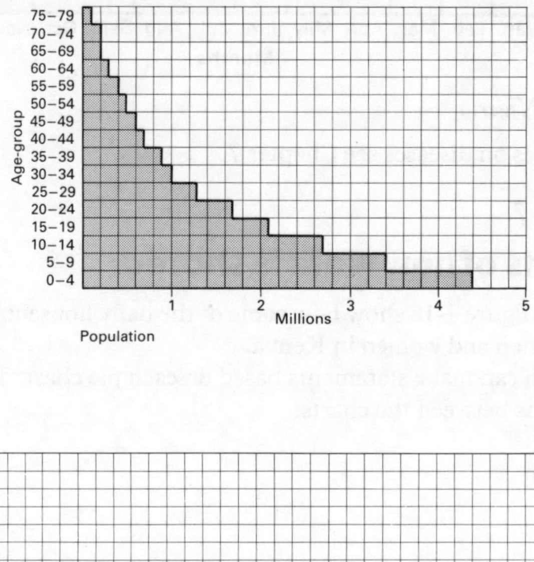

(b)

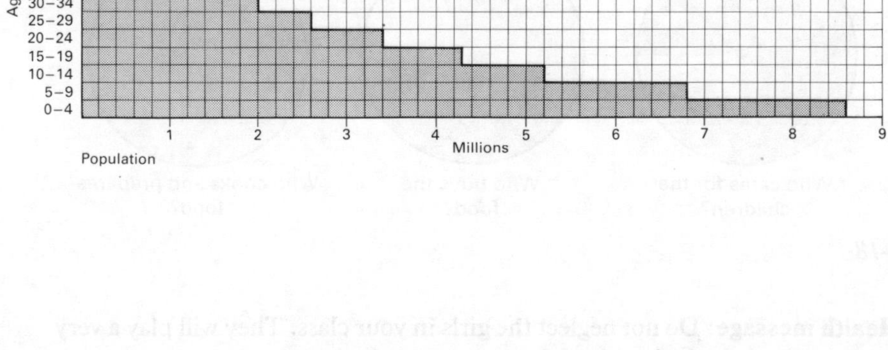

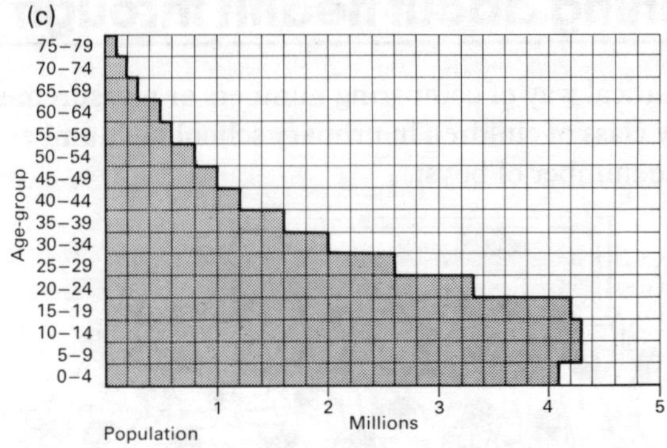

1-19 Population pyramids: (a) for Kenya in 1985 with family size of 8 children per mother (b) for Kenya in year 2000 (no change in family size) (c) for Kenya in year 2000 with family size of 4 children per mother

The children can compare the charts and make deductions.

For more activities on population see Chapter 5.

2 Teaching about health through ratios

Ratio is a mathematical way of comparing numbers or measurements. For example, with any class of children in primary school the number of girls can be compared with the number of boys.

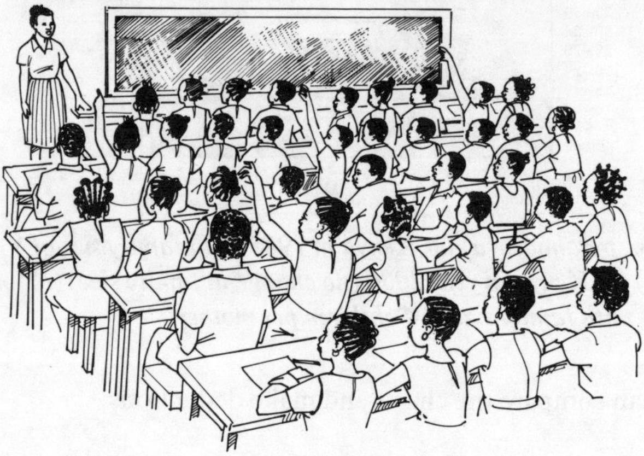

2-1

Look at this picture of a primary school class (figure 2-1). The ratio of girls to boys is 16 : 21.

In the same way any two measurements can be compared as long as the units used for both are the same.

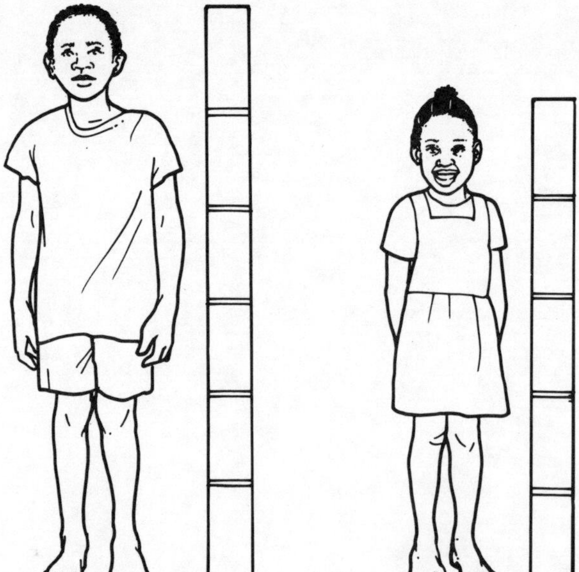

2-2

The ratio of Muthoni's height to Ngugi's is 5 : 6.

Here are some simple ratio activities connected with the main health themes.

• Activity 1 — Middle
• Sex ratios

The children can find out the ratio of male population to female population

- in their own family, including mother, father and their brothers and sisters,
- in their own household,
- in their own class,
- in their own school,
- in their own group (see page 24),
- in their own nation.

Remember that:

- ratio is always given simply as numbers 2 : 3 *not* 2 boys : 3 girls.
- the order of the numbers is the same as the order of the sentence;
  ratio of Muthoni's height to Ngugi's height is 5 : 6
  ratio of Ngugi's height to Muthoni's height is 6 : 5
- ratio can be simplified
  3 : 12 is the same as 1 : 4.
- ratio is not ration.

For more activities on population see Chapter 5.

• Activity 2 — Middle
• Health ratios in the class

The children in the class can each carry out their own survey. Each child chooses a simple question about health to ask the rest of the class. Here are some questions they might ask:

Have you ever had a tooth that hurt?
Have you had measles?
Have you ever broken a bone?
Have you ever drunk poison by mistake?
Do you ever help with the cooking?
Have you a BCG scar?

Each child then asks all the others in the class the question.
All those who answer 'yes' have a tick ✓ put beside their name.
All those who answer 'no' have a cross × put beside their name.
When all have answered, the ratio of 'yes' to 'no' answers can be worked out.

Example: Absy asked the whole class if they had ever had a cut that needed treatment in the dispensary. 10 answered 'yes', 32 answered 'no'. Absy then wrote: 'The ratio of children who have had a cut treated at the dispensary to those who have not is 10 : 32 or 5 : 16.

Children can make a *ratio facts* chart about their class.

A practical note about simplifying ratios

The number of children in your class will determine whether or not the ratios from class surveys will simplify. For example, if there are 24 children in your class then many of the possible results will simplify.

Survey results that will simplify:

2 : 22 becomes 1 : 11
3 : 21 becomes 1 : 7
4 : 20 becomes 1 : 5
6 : 18 becomes 1 : 3
8 : 16 becomes 1 : 2
9 : 15 becomes 3 : 5
10 : 14 becomes 5 : 7
12 : 12 becomes 1 : 1

Survey results that will not simplify:

1 : 23
5 : 19
7 : 17
11 : 13

Many results from a class of 24 will simplify because 24 has many factors. If you have 23 in the class then no results will simplify as 23 is a prime number.

If your class size has many factors (e.g. 36, 30, 32), then many of the results from the class survey will simplify. If your class size does not have many factors, then either include yourself in the survey, for example,

47 children + 1 teacher = 48 (this has many factors)

or leave out the child making the survey, for example,

43 children − 1 child = 42 (this also has many factors).

By using either of these tactics you will find that the class survey activity will lead to more ratios that can be simplified.

Comparing ratios

One of the main uses of ratios is to compare two situations. For example, in Malu School there are 8 teachers and 240 pupils. In Dambwa School there are 21 teachers and 672 pupils. Which school is better off for teachers?

The ratio of teachers to pupils in the two schools can be found (see Table 2-1).

Table 2-1

School	Ratio of teachers to pupils	Simplified ratio
Malu	8 : 240	1 : 30
Dambwa	21 : 672	1 : 32

By comparing the two ratios we can see that Malu School is better supplied with teachers than Dambwa school.

The numbers in this example were chosen carefully so that the ratios were easily simplified. If the numbers come from real surveys carried out by the children then the numbers will often be harder to work with.

For example, Seth carried out a survey of BCG immunization in two households. His results are shown in figure 2-3.

	Children immunized	Children not immunized
Household A	5	12
Household B	4	9

2-3

To compare the two households each ratio is reduced to a unit ratio.

Household A 5 : 12 becomes $1 : \frac{12}{5}$ or 1 : 2.4

Household B 4 : 9 becomes $1 : \frac{9}{4}$ or 1 : 2.25

Now the two households can be compared. Household B has taken better care of its children.

For more activities on immunization see Chapter 7.

• Activity 3 Middle

• Sanitation ratios

The children can find out the ratio of those in the class who

- have latrines to those who do not,
- boil their drinking water to those who do not,
- cover their water storage to those who do not.

The children can calculate the ratio of latrines to pupils in their school and then compare this ratio with the official recommended ratio. The children should

- find out the total number of latrines the children use in the school,
- find out the number of children in the school,
- find the ratio of latrines to children,
- then compare their school ratio with the official recommended ratio.

Example:

Table 2-2

School	Number of latrines	Number of pupils
Shingu	5	280
Chinga	12	360

In Shingu School the ratio of latrines to pupils is 5 : 280 or 1: 56.
In Chinga School the ratio of latrines to pupils is 12 : 360 or 1 : 30.

The official recommendation in Kenya is that there should be 1 latrine for every 40 pupils. Which school should build more latrines?

For more activities on sanitation see Chapter 9.

• Activity 4 Upper

• Age ratios

One of the striking facts about African populations is the high ratio of young to old. Here are some ways for children to study this ratio.

- Children can carry out a survey of their home and find the ratio of those under 15 years old to those over 15 years.
- Children can compare their own home ratio with the ratios found by other children in the class.
- Children can compare their home ratio with the national ratio.

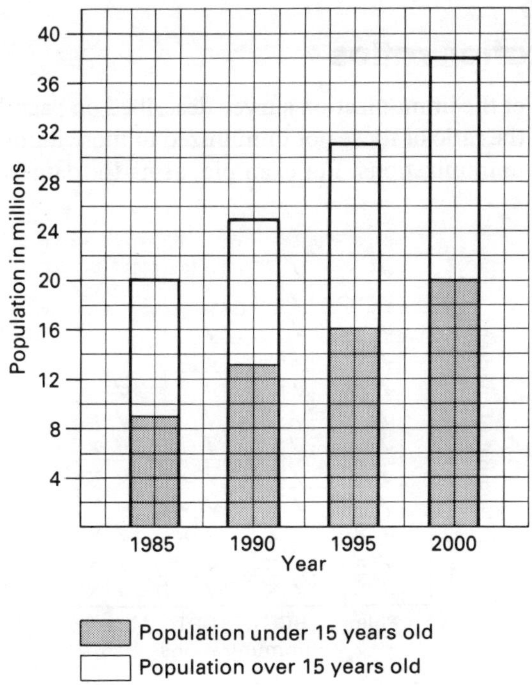

2-4 Population in Kenya between 1985 and the year 2000

The information needed can be found from the graph in Figure 2-4. The population under 15 years old is shown by the shaded section of the column. For example, in 1985

Population under 15 = 9 million
Population over 15 = 11 million

Ratio of under 15's to over 15's

9 : 11
or 1 : 1.2 (to one decimal place)

Using the predicted populations shown on the graph the children can work out the same ratio for future years.

For more activities on population see Chapter 5.

• Activity 5 Upper

• Immunization ratios

Using the results of the immunization survey described on page 111, the children can find the ratio of those not immunized to those immunized for each of the four major immunizations. For example, using the data from the chart in figure 2-5:

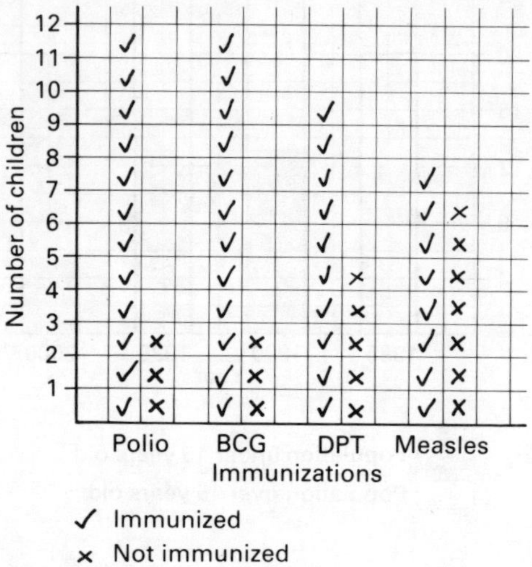

2-5 Chart of a class immunization survey

For polio: ratio of those not immunized to those immunized

3 : 12
or 1 : 4

For more activities on immunization see Chapter 7.

• Activity 6 Upper

• Body ratios

Finding the ratios of the lengths of various parts of the body provides an interesting exercise. The units used will make no difference to the resulting ratio as long as the same unit is used for both measures. So the ratio can be found using arbitrary units of the children's choice as well as using standard units.

Here are some ideas.

- The children can measure the height of their navel and their total height then find the ratio between the two distances.

- The children can find the ratio of stretch to height.

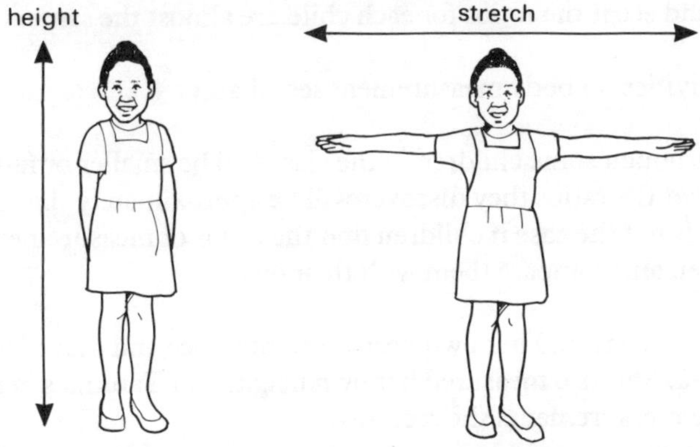

- The children can find the ratio of sitting height to standing height.

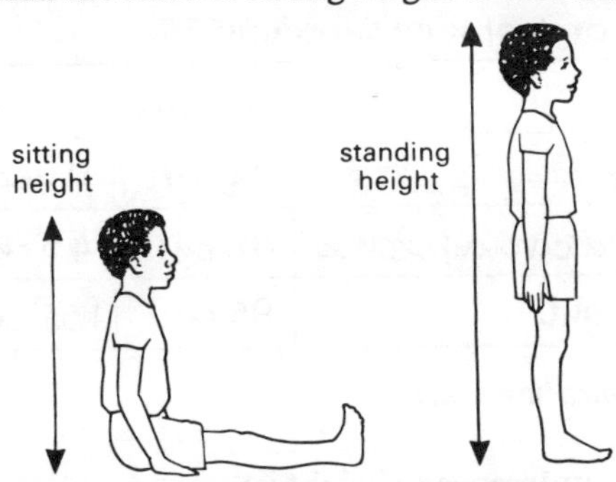

2-6

- The children can measure the distance around their wrists (Plate 2), around their necks and around their waists. They can compare these distances using ratios.

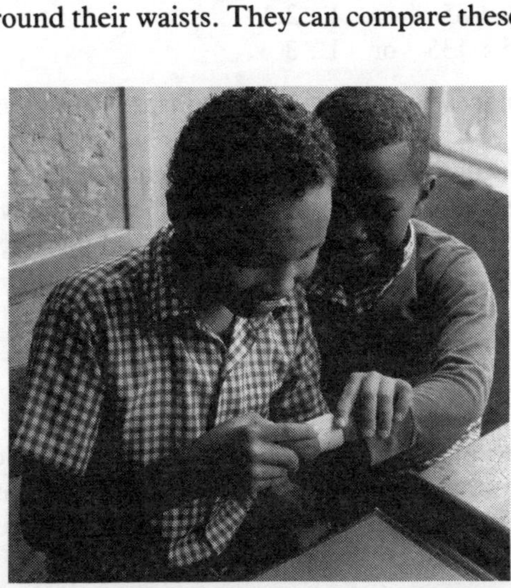

Plate 2 Measuring wrist circumference

- The children decide on two lengths of their own body which they wish to compare and see if the ratios for each child are almost the same.

For more activities on body measurement see Chapter 4.

In general, although some children in the class will be smaller or fatter than others, many of the ratios they discover will be approximately the same.

But this is not the case if children find the ratios of measurements for very young children and compare them with their own.

Example: Mary measured her own head circumference and that of her young sister, Tabitha. She also measured her own height and Tabitha's height. Figure 2-7 shows the measurements she recorded.

Record of measurements

	Tabitha	Mary
Age	2 years	11 years
Head circumference	40 cm	45 cm
Height	85 cm	135 cm

2-7 Mary's record of measurements

The ratio of head circumference to height is:

for Tabitha 40 : 85 or 1 : 2.1
for Mary 45 : 135 or 1 : 3

Encourage the children to measure their younger brothers and sisters and work out ratios.

The children will find that the ratios in young children are different. The proportions of their bodies are not the same. The head grows very rapidly after birth and will be almost fully grown by the time a child is five years old. The rest of the body will not be fully grown until the age of 18 or 19.

• Activity 7 Upper

• Sugar–salt solution

When a sugar–salt solution is made up to give to those with diarrhoea it is important that the amounts mixed are in the correct ratio (see page 124).

If the paper cups made from 3 cm and 6 cm squares are used then the solution is made like this:

Small paper cup of salt + larger paper cup of sugar for 1 glass of water

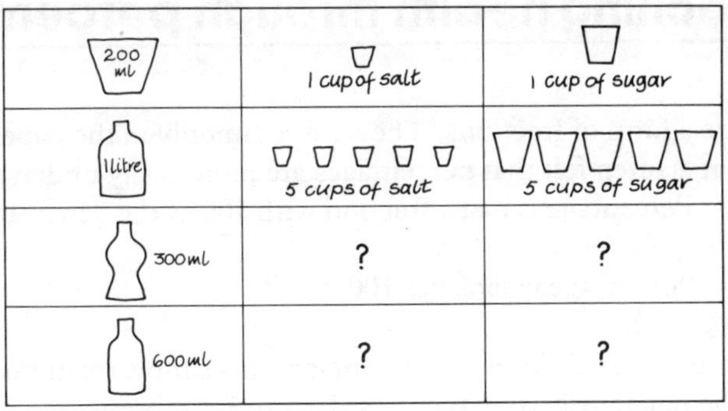

2-8

- The children can bring bottles of many different sizes to school. Nearly all will have their capacity marked on them.
- The children can build up a table like the one in figure 2-8 to show how many cups of salt and sugar should be added to each bottle to give the correct strength of solution.
- The children can also find the ratio of the volume of the salt cup to the sugar cup.

  First they should make paper cups: one from a 3 cm square, the other from a 6 cm square. (Instructions are given in figure 8-7 on page 128.)

  The children can discover how many of the small cups will fill the large cup by filling them using sand.

  It should take about 8 salt cups to fill the sugar cup, so the ratio of the volumes will be 1 : 8.

This activity is an excellent practical way of developing a difficult mathematical concept.

The ratio of the lengths of the paper squares is 3 : 6 or 1 : 2
The ratio of the areas of the paper squares is 9 : 36 or 1 : 4
The ratio of the volumes of the paper cups made from the squares was 1 : 8

The children can find the ratios when the salt cup is compared with a cup made from a 9 cm square.

For more activities on the sugar–salt solution see Chapter 8.

3 Teaching health through percentage

Percentages are a form of fractions. They are commonly in the papers and on the radio because it is often felt that percentages are more easily understood than other fractions. Percentage is just a fraction with 100 as the denominator.

$\frac{23}{100} = 23\%$ Percentage means per 100.

When introducing children to percentage, this simple relationship with fractions can be put across using pictures. Figure 3-1 represents

$\frac{37}{100}$ or 37%

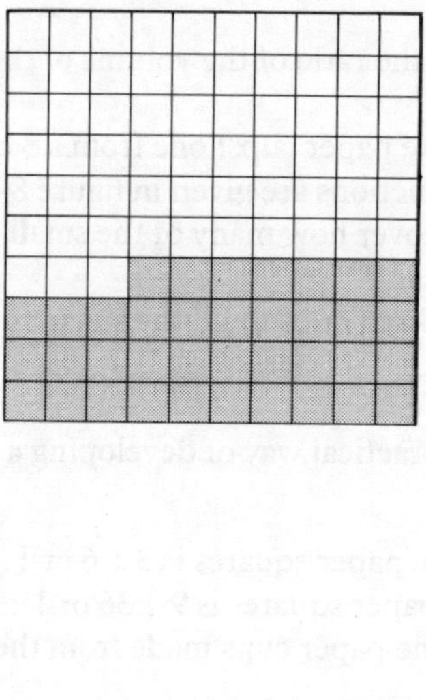

3-1

• Activity 1 Middle

• Disease survey of 100 children

To create percentage pictures, the children can draw around a 10 by 10 square on squared paper.

The children then carry out a survey of 100 children (this can be done during break time). For example, they ask 100 children if they have had measles. Each child's answer is recorded in a square: a tick for 'yes' and a cross for 'no' (see figure 3-2).

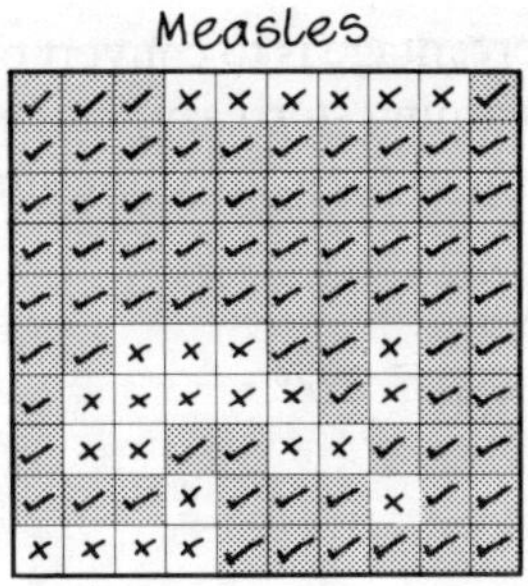

3-2

The children can then colour over all the ticks and find the total number of ticks out of 100. They can write this both as a fraction and as a percentage:

$\frac{74}{100}$ have had measles   74% have had measles.

Some examples of other surveys carried out by children in this way are shown in figure 3-3.

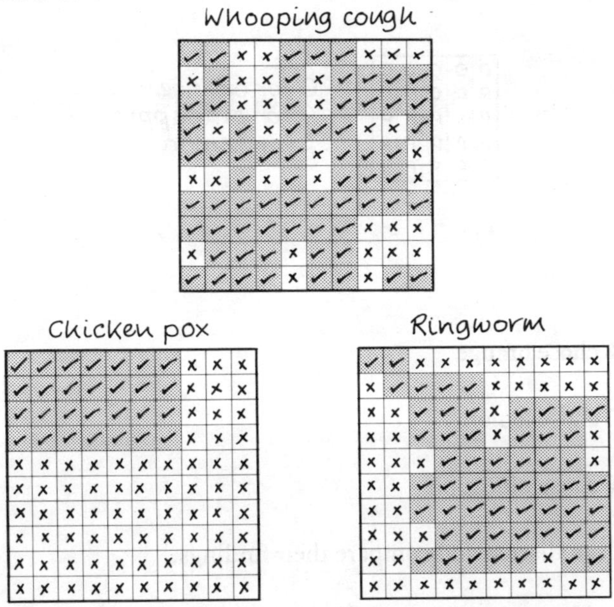

3-3

The children can compare the percentages discovered in the surveys and find which disease is most common. Using the charts shown here

- 67% have had whooping cough,
- 28% have had chicken pox,
- 55% have had ringworm.

For more activities on infectious diseases see Chapter 7.

The next stage in teaching percentage is to convert other fractions to percentages. To make each learning step easy, move next to fractions with 50, 25, 20 or 10 as the denominator as these are quite simple to change to percentages.

$$\frac{17}{50} = \frac{34}{100} = 34\% \quad \text{or} \quad \frac{9}{25} = \frac{36}{100} = 36\%$$

• Activity 2 Middle

• Survey of 25 children's favourite fruits

The children can prepare a 5 by 5 square marked on squared paper.

The children choose three of the Go, Glow or Grow fruits (see page 98) and ask 25 of their classmates to pick their favourite. They show each answer by a different symbol (figure 3-4).

The children find the percentage who chose each fruit.

O	O	O	O	O
P	L	O	O	O
P	L	P	P	P
P	P	P	P	P
P	P	P	P	P

O for orange
P for pineapple
L for lemon

3-4

Example:

$\frac{8}{25}$ or 32% chose orange

$\frac{2}{25}$ or 8% chose lemon

$\frac{15}{25}$ or 60% chose pineapple

The children can discuss and compare their findings.

For more activities on nutrition see Chapter 6.

• Activity 3 Middle

• Accident survey of 20 children

The children can choose which accident they would like to survey. Each can pick a different one and ask 20 others in the class if they have ever had that accident.

The chart in figure 3-5 shows the results of a child who made a survey of whether or not children had been badly cut and needed stitches.

How many had stitches?

Badly cut and needed stitches

✓	✓	✓	×	×
✓	✓	×	×	×
×	×	×	×	×
×	×	×	×	×

$$\frac{5}{20} = 25\%$$

3-5

For more activities on accidents see Chapter 1.

• Activity 4 — Middle/upper

• From tenths to percentages

This activity gives children practice in changing from fractions out of ten straight to percentages, for example, from $\frac{7}{10}$ to 70%.

Group the class in sets of ten. (Some children may have to be left out so that each group has just ten members. These children can act as recorders or as monitors to make sure each group answers questions honestly.) Ask each group to find out how many in the group are right-handed. The answer should then be given as a percentage. For example, if 9 out of 10 in the group are right-handed the answer given by the group will be: 90% of our group are right-handed.

Here are some further questions you can ask each group:

What percentage of children in your group
- eat eggs?
- can put their arm over their head and touch their ear?
- have a scar on their hand or arm?
- have clean finger nails?
- can curl their tongue?
- have white teeth?
- can wiggle their ears?
- have combed their hair?
- are over 1 metre tall?
- can grip all the way around their wrist?
- have no sisters?
- have a loose tooth?
- fold their arms right-over-left?
- can touch their toes without bending their knees?

Choose the questions that you feel are suitable or make up some of your own that relate to health issues.

• Activity 5 Upper
• The class survey

It is very likely that the number of children in your class is not a factor of 100. If it is 50, 25 or 20, then children are easily able to convert the results of class surveys to percentages. But if it is 37 or 41 for example, then these are difficult numbers with which to calculate. To help children convert the results of class surveys to percentages they can make a *class percentage conversion chart*. The example in figure 3-6 is for a class of 33 children.

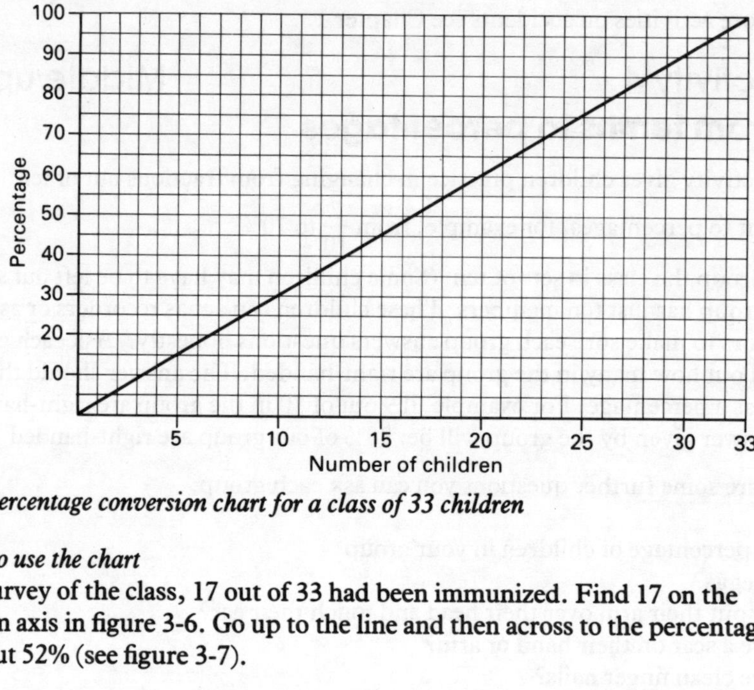

3-6 Percentage conversion chart for a class of 33 children

How to use the chart

In a survey of the class, 17 out of 33 had been immunized. Find 17 on the bottom axis in figure 3-6. Go up to the line and then across to the percentage. It is about 52% (see figure 3-7).

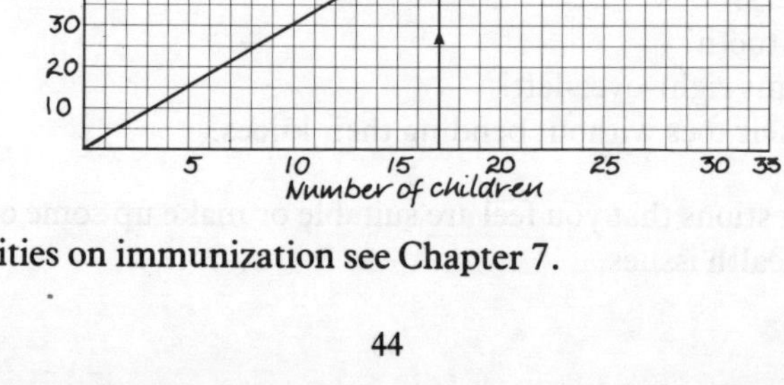

3-7

For more activities on immunization see Chapter 7.

The children can carry out surveys on a variety of health topics and convert their findings to percentages.

If there is more than one stream in your school, encourage each class to carry out the same health surveys and compare the results. See, for example, the survey of 3 standard 6 classes, P, R and S in figure 3-8.

Percentage of children	Standard 6 P	Standard 6 R	Standard 6 S
who have had severe burns	17%	10%	15%
who know how to make a sugar-salt solution	83%	7%	40%
who are over 1·5 metres in height	56%	61%	59%
who regularly eat 'Glow' foods	75%	30%	29%
who have been immunized against measles	88%	80%	73%
with proper sanitation at home	64%	47%	86%

3-8

Using percentages to compare

One of the main reasons for using percentages and not ordinary fractions is that percentages are easy to compare.

For example, 13 out of 50 children have had measles in class A. In another class B, 6 out of 24 have had measles.

$\frac{13}{50}$ and $\frac{6}{24}$ are not easy to compare.

If both fractions are changed to a percentage then they become 26% and 25%. Class A has the higher percentage.

• Activity 6 — Upper
• Comparing percentages

Here is some data connected with health. In order to compare and make a judgement about the data, it has to be changed to percentages.

Example: Out of 80 babies who were breast-fed, 8 died in the first year. Out of 60 babies fed on bottle milk, 18 died in the first year.

What percentage of breast-fed babies died? What percentage of bottle-fed babies died? Which is healthier for babies, breast or bottle?

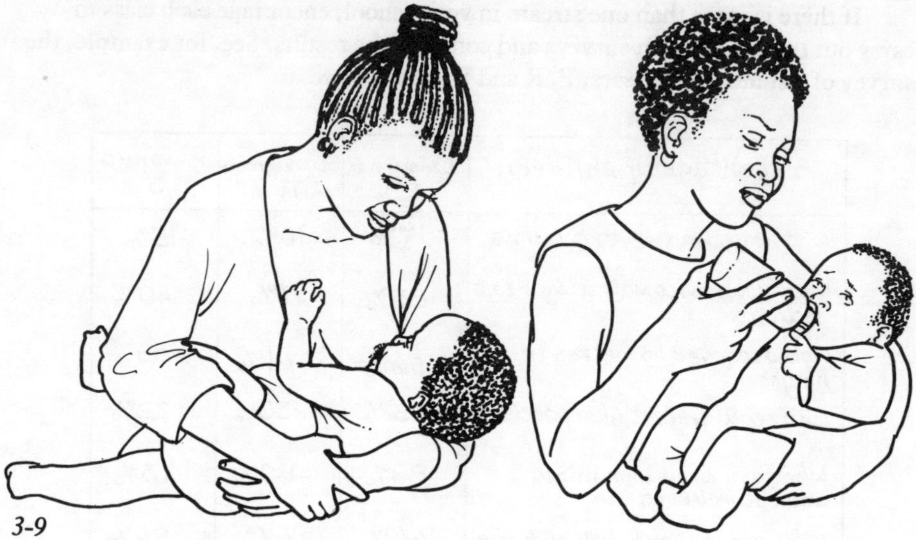

3-9

Percentage of breast-fed babies dying in 1st year $= \frac{8}{80} \times 100 = 10\%$

Percentage of bottle-fed babies dying in 1st year $= \frac{18}{60} \times 100 = 30\%$

Now it is easy to decide which method of feeding babies is best. This is why many health workers use the phrase 'breast is best'! It is clear that the percentage of bottle-fed babies dying in the first year is much higher.

For more activities on breast feeding see Chapter 6.

• Activity 7 — Upper

• Birth rate

A very rough way to find birth rate is to ask your class how many of them have a baby brother or sister under one year old. The children can then calculate this as a percentage. For example, in a class of 40, 10 of the children have a baby brother or sister under one year old.

Birth rate $= \frac{10}{40} \times 100\% = 25\%$

(The birth rate found in this way will be much higher than the national birth rate. Can you think why?)

National birth rates

The children can now study the birth rates in different countries. Ask the children to look at Table 3-1 and

- compare the birth rates in different countries,
- find countries with the same birth rate,
- find the country with the lowest birth rate.

Table 3-1

Country	Birth rate
Malawi	5%
Zambia	5%
Gabon	3%
Ghana	5%
Uganda	5%
Tanzania	5%
Lesotho	4%
Kenya	5%

The children can then do some calculations using the percentages in the table.

Exercise
Here is a list of villages in different countries and the population of each village. Using Table 3-1, can you work out how many babies are likely to be born in each village next year?

Mbusyani in Kenya has a population of 900
Namashakende in Zambia has a population of 400
Motu in Lesotho has a population of 500
Terani in Gabon has a population of 300

Example: In Lesotho the birth rate is 4%, so the number of babies that are likely to be born in Motu is

$$\frac{4}{100} \times 500 = 20 \text{ babies}$$

For more activities on population see Chapter 5.

- Activity 8 **Upper**
- **Infant death rate**

One way of measuring the health of a village, a province or a country is to work out the *infant death rate*. This rate is found by calculating the percentage of babies who die before they are one year old. You will probably feel that it is wrong for children to collect statistics on infant deaths from their homes. Instead you might like to introduce the idea through a story.

The wise chief

In a certain village on the side of a great mountain lived a chief who cared greatly for all his people. One day the chief decided that he would keep a record of all the children born in the village. He called all the people together and told them that each time a baby was born the chief would plant a fruit tree on the hillside. And so it happened. Every time a baby was born, the chief planted a new tree. At the end of a year the chief had planted 40 trees. He called all the villagers together and asked each mother to place her baby beside one of the fruit trees. But when this was done there were 8 trees that had no babies beside them. 'Where are the babies?' the chief asked. 'They have died' the sad mothers replied. Then the chief called all his counsellors together. He asked them 'What percentage of the babies born this year have died?'

At this point, ask the children to calculate this percentage, which is called the *infant death rate*.

Babies dying in first year = 8
Number of babies = 40

Infant death rate $= \frac{8}{40} \times 100\% = 20\%$

Then the chief asked 'Is our village a healthy village?'

Table 3-2

Country	**Infant death rate**
Malawi	16%
Sierra Leone	18%
Burundi	12%
Nigeria	11%
Tanzania	11%
Uganda	11%
Ghana	9%
Zambia	8%
Kenya	8%
Zimbabwe	8%

Now ask the children to look at the infant death rates in many different countries (Table 3-2).

Ask them to compare the rates in the different countries.
Ask them to compare the rate in the story with the rates shown here.
How would they answer the chief's question?

Then the chief asked his counsellors 'Why are the babies dying? How can we make our village a healthier one?'

Ask the children what answers they would give. This will give you a chance to discuss with the class the major causes of death among young children and the action that children can take to fight the death rate.

Table 3-3

Causes	**Actions**
Malnutrition	Breast feed babies
	After 4 months give extra food
Diarrhoea	Clean water
	Good latrines
	The sugar–salt solution
Measles and tetanus	Make sure babies are immunized

A note to teachers
In this section we have talked about the *infant death rate*. In most handbooks of national statistics this is usually called the *Infant Mortality Rate (IMR)* and is measured in deaths per thousand. Here deaths per *hundred* has been used to link the work with percentages.

For more activities on population see Chapter 5.

PART B

Mathematics into health

4 Body and growth measurement

Measuring children regularly is a sensitive way to check that they are growing well. To keep a clear record of each child's growth many health clinics now use a growth chart.

Each child has his/her own growth chart kept by the mother. Each month the mother brings the child and the chart to the clinic. The child is weighed and the weight is recorded on the chart.

As the chart is filled month by month it gives a graph of the child's growth. If the child is growing well then the graph will follow a steadily rising path and will lie between the two lines shown on the chart in figure 4-1(a).

(a)

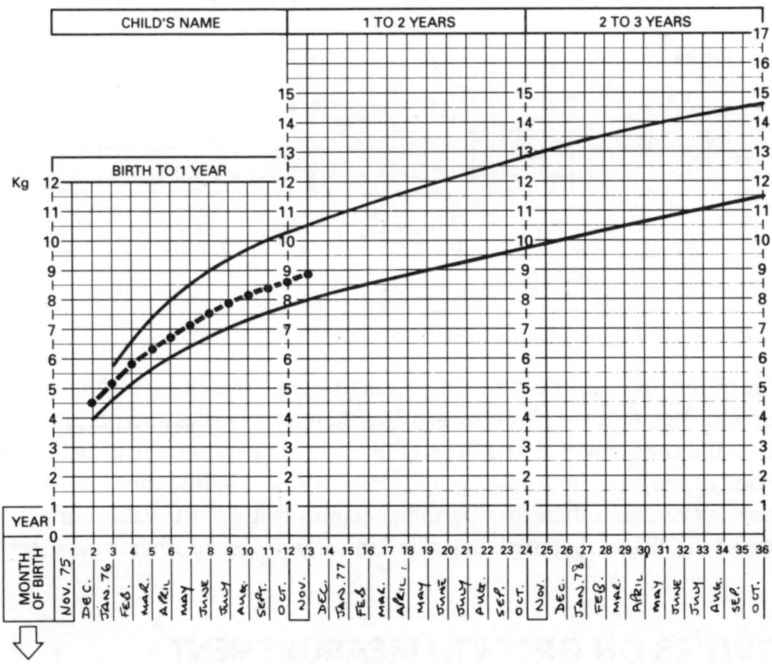

4-1 (a) The growth chart of a healthy baby

The two lines show the range within which most children's weights should lie. If the child is not growing well then the graph may look like figure 4-1(b).

This age/weight graph, or 'growth chart' as it is called, is not easy for primary school children or their parents to understand. Yet the growth chart is very important in the drive for improved health care. The health chart can warn the health worker or parent if a baby is not growing properly and action can quickly be taken to prevent further ill health.

(b)

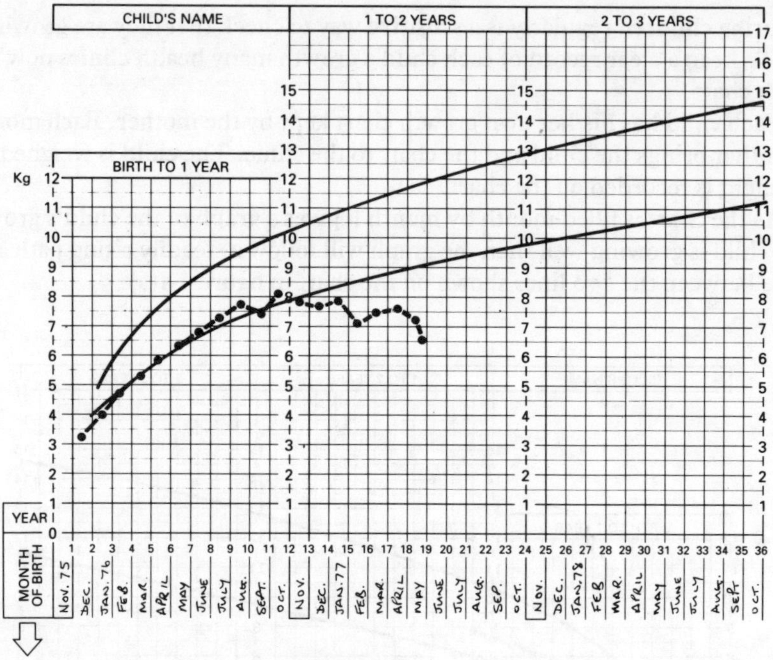

4-1 (b) The growth chart of a sick baby

One of the main aims of this chapter is to suggest teaching activities which will help children to learn about measuring their own bodies and prepare them to understand the growth chart. When they become parents, the growth chart will be one of the most important graphs they will see. While they are still children they can help their own parents become aware of the value and meaning of the charts that are being filled in for younger brothers and sisters.

ACTIVITIES ON GROWTH MEASUREMENT

Most schools do not have scales for measuring the weight of children. So the practical activities in this chapter concentrate on measuring height and developing the idea of the age–height graph.

The age–height graph (figure 4-2) is very similar to the age–weight graph. Drawing and using the age–height graph can be done in any primary school classroom and children will then find it easier to understand the age–weight graph.

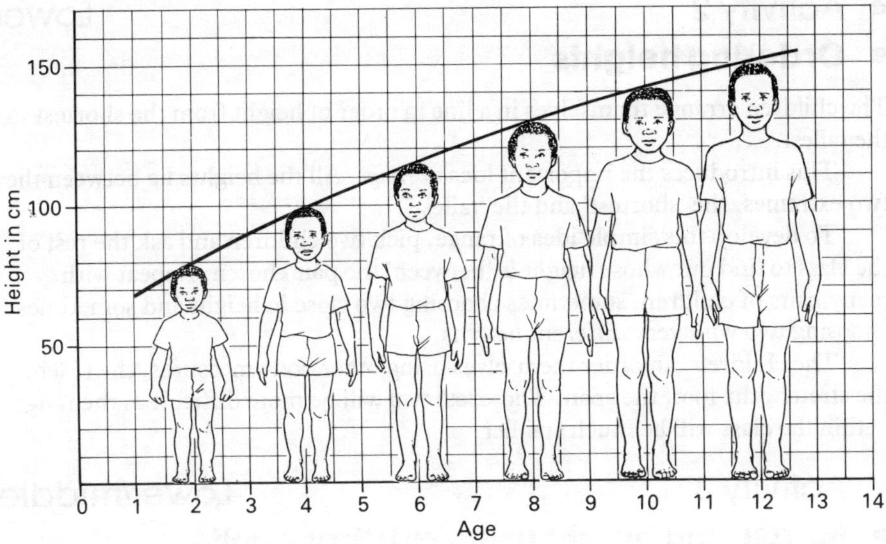

4-2 The age–height graph

• Activity 1 — Lower

• Comparing heights

Choose one child of middle height to stand in front of the class. Let the other children come one by one and stand back-to-back with the chosen child. They can then say 'I am taller than Mary' or 'I am shorter than Mary' or 'I am the same height as Mary.' You can then choose other children to be the standard against whom the others are compared.

Let the children compare other parts of their bodies by direct comparison. For example,

their reach
their stretch
their span
their feet

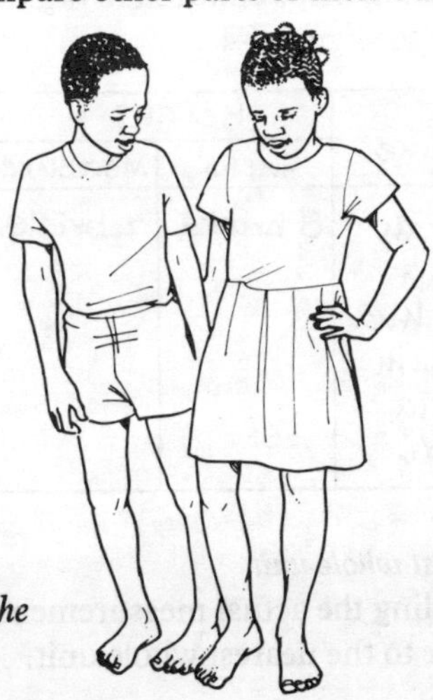

4-3 Children comparing the size of their feet

• Activity 2 — Lower

• Ordering heights

The children arrange themselves in a line in order of height from the shortest to the tallest.

This introduces the important idea of *range*. All the heights lie between the two extremes, the 'shortest' and the 'tallest'.

To develop this simple idea of range, pick two children and ask the rest of the class to find out whose height is 'between' the pair chosen. Repeat with many pairs of children, sometimes choosing two close in height and sometimes choosing two with very different heights.

The children can order themselves using other body measures, the reach, the stretch, the foot, the span. These last two will be more difficult as the range within the class will be much smaller.

• Activity 3 — Lower/middle

• Measuring height using arbitrary units

Before measuring with the standard units, metres and centimetres, which are rather too large or too small respectively, introduce the children to measuring using objects of their choice.

For example, they can measure their height in bricks or exercise books or using their own hand-span.

At this stage encourage two important mathematical skills:

(a) *Estimation or 'good guessing'*
When the children are making a table for their results, always have a column in which the children can put their guess. Make sure they guess before measuring. Guessing helps children to build a mental picture of the unit used in measuring (see figure 4-4).

Name	Height	
	Guess	Measure
Sarah	8 bricks	7 bricks
John		
Joshua		
Salim		
Faria		
Abdi		

4-4

(b) *Measurement to the nearest whole unit*
In the column for recording the actual measurement, the children should learn to fill in the answer to the nearest whole unit.

The children can now measure other parts of their bodies using units of their own choice, for example,

measuring span using matchsticks
measuring feet using bottle-tops
measuring noses using finger tips

• Activity 4 Middle

• Measuring using metric units

Let the children measure each other against a height chart marked in centimetres on the wall as in figure 4-5. Once again encourage them to guess the height before measuring.

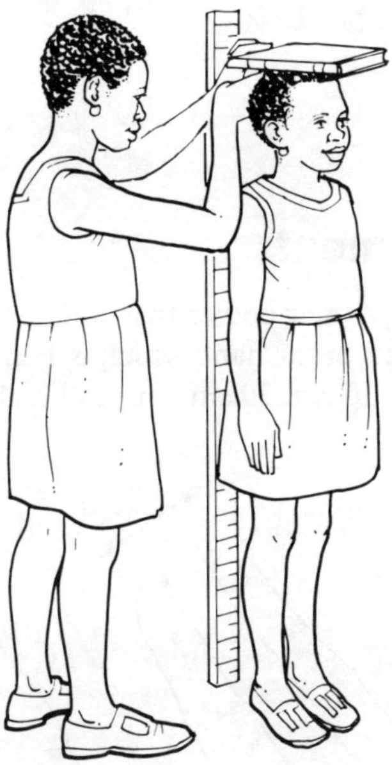

4-5

A valuable exercise in subtraction is to ask the children to calculate the difference in height between various pairs.

The greatest difference in heights will be between the shortest and tallest in the class and will give the range of heights in the class.

Tallest in class	=	126 cm
Shortest in class	=	104 cm
Range	=	22 cm

The children can measure other parts of the body using standard units. For example,

the reach
the stretch
the span
the hand
the little finger
the foot

- The children can find the class range for each of these parts of the body.
- The children can measure the parts of the body of their younger brothers and sisters and make a record of their findings (see figure 4-6).

Body chart of my brother, age 5	Height = Reach = Stretch =	Little finger = Hand = Foot =

4-6

• Activity 5 Upper
• Body measurements

Let the children find parts of their bodies that will be useful for measuring. For example, can they find a part of the hand which is 1 cm wide or long? Let them find some part that is 5 cm, 10 cm, 20 cm long and make up a table. For example,

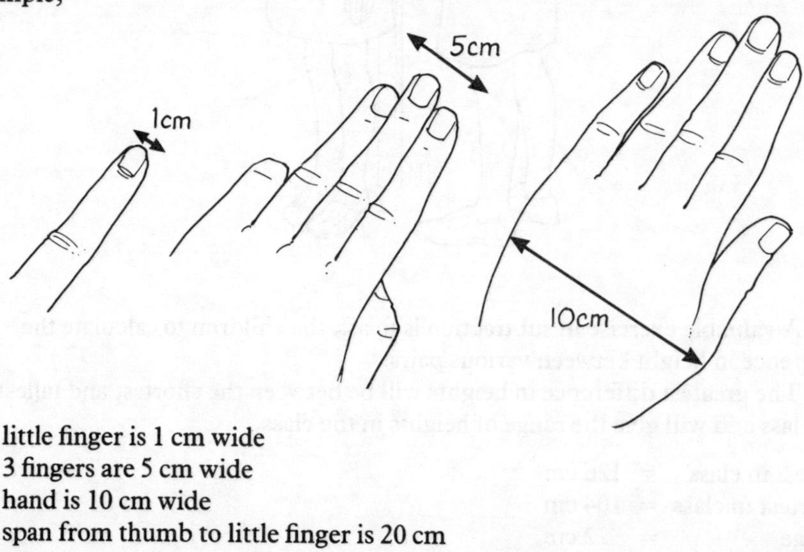

4-7

my little finger is 1 cm wide
my 3 fingers are 5 cm wide
my hand is 10 cm wide
my span from thumb to little finger is 20 cm

• Activity 6 Middle/upper

• Measuring around parts of the body

Measuring around objects is harder than measuring in a straight line. The idea that a curved line, when straightened, does not change its length, is not obvious to young children and needs plenty of first-hand experience.

Even adults are very poor at estimating the length around objects, they nearly always give an answer which is too small.

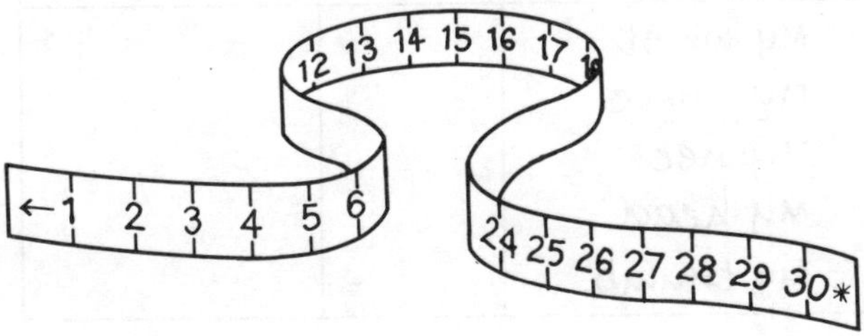

4-8 The measuring strip

Each child can make a measuring strip from a piece of paper or thin card. The strip should be about 2 cm wide and 30 cm long (see figure 4-8). The strip is marked in centimetres with an ← showing zero centimetres and a * at the other end.

The children place the * end of the strip on a tin. The strip is then wrapped around the tin (see figure 4-9).

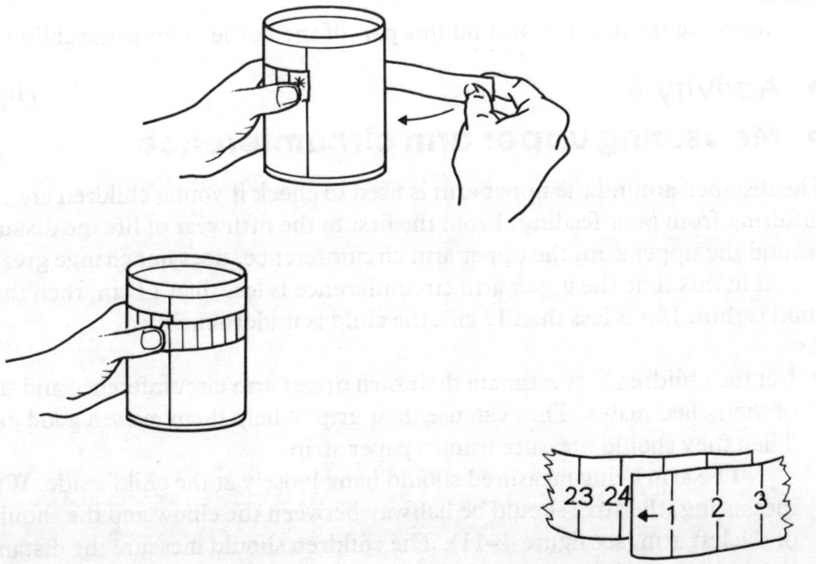

4-9

The children look at the arrow and find the mark to which it is nearest. This gives the distance around the tin, to the nearest centimetre.

The children can practise on tins, bottles and sticks. The children can then measure around parts of their body and record the answers in a table like the one in figure 4-10.

Table of measurement

Distance around	Guess	Measure
My wrist		
My ankle		
My neck		
My head		
My thumb		

4-10

• Activity 7 Middle/upper

• Measuring grip

The grip is not easy to measure. Here is one way.

Can the child's fingers touch around the top of a bottle? Can they touch around the middle of the bottle? Find the place where the child's fingers just touch.

Measure the distance around this part of the bottle. This is the child's *grip*.

• Activity 8 Upper

• Measuring upper arm circumference

The distance around the upper arm is used to check if young children are suffering from poor feeding. From the first to the fifth year of life the distance around the upper arm, the upper arm circumference, does not change greatly.

If in this time the upper arm circumference is less than 13 cm, then the child is thin. If it is less than 12 cm, the child is undernourished.

- Let the children first estimate their own upper arm circumference and those of their class mates. They can use their grip to help them make a good guess. Then they should measure using a paper strip.

  The arm being measured should hang loosely at the child's side. When measuring, the strip should be halfway between the elbow and the shoulder of the left arm (see figure 4–11). The children should measure the distance to the nearest centimetre.

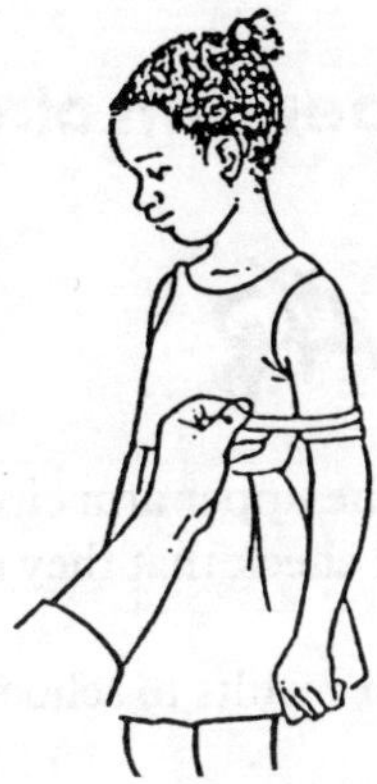

4-11

- **The children can measure the upper arm circumference of the youngest children in the school, the 'standard one' children or those in the pre-unit. They should measure to the nearest centimetre and keep a record of their results (figure 4–12).**

Distance around upper arm

Name	Guess	Measure
Kari		
Amali		

4-12

The children can make a chart of all the measurements they have made as shown in figure 4-13.

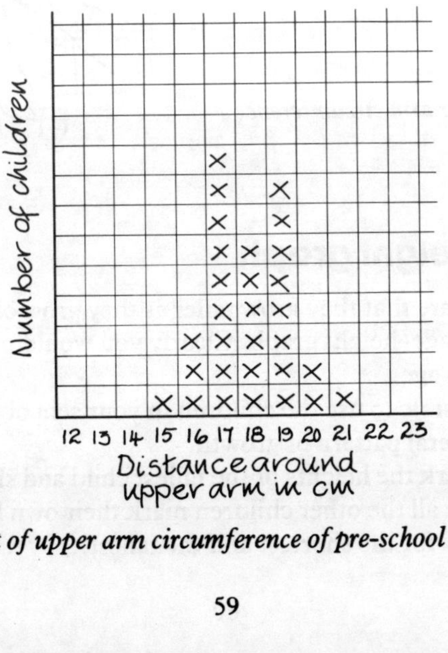

4-13 Children's chart of upper arm circumference of pre-school children

• Activity 9 Upper

• Measuring the upper arm circumference of younger children

The children can now measure the upper arm circumference of their younger brothers and sisters at home and check that they are not malnourished (see figure 4-14).

The children can bring their results to school so that you can talk with the children about them in class.

As a teacher you have to decide on the most tactful way to deal with any measurements that suggest cases of malnourishment. First have the measurement checked, then either talk to the parents confidentially or pass the information on to the health clinic. (See also Chapter 5 Activity 6)

Remember that any child between 1 and 5 years old whose upper arm circumference is 13 cm is thin and may well be undernourished. A child with a measurement of 12 cm or less is certainly malnourished. (See also Chapter 6, Activity 6.)

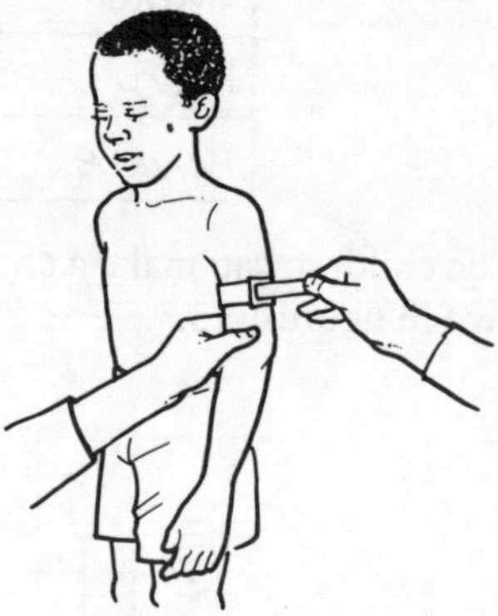

4-14 Measuring upper arm circumference

• Activity 10 Upper

• The age–height graph

Children are well aware that they grow taller as they grow older but it is not practical to make an age–height graph. Clearly you would need a record of the child's height at each age.

Instead it is possible to use the children in your school to make a graph which shows the general pattern of growth.

In your class mark the heights of the tallest child and shortest child on the blackboard. Then let all the other children mark their own heights. They will lie in between the marks for the shortest and the tallest.

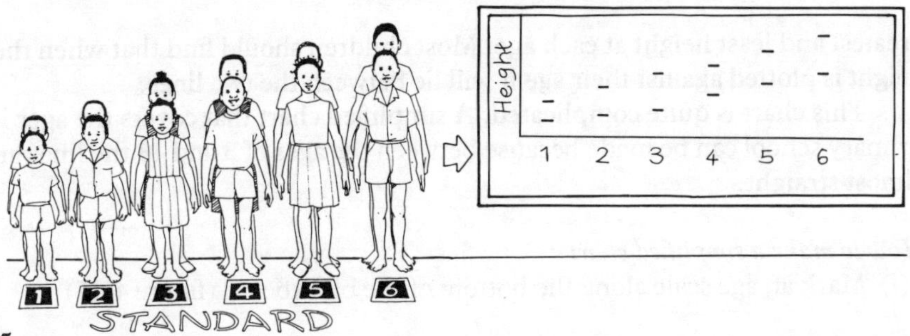

4-15

Now ask the children to find the shortest and tallest child in each standard in the school (this will take a little bit of organization and cooperation with other teachers). The children then mark the heights of these children in columns on the board. This will give a 'road' of growth between which all children in the school will lie (see figure 4-15).

A warning: This activity assumes that children in each standard are very similar in age. If your school has children of many different ages in each standard then find the shortest and tallest of each age to make the chart.

• Activity 11 Upper

• The age-height chart

The heights of many children at different ages have been measured. These measurements have been used to make the chart in figure 4-16 which shows the

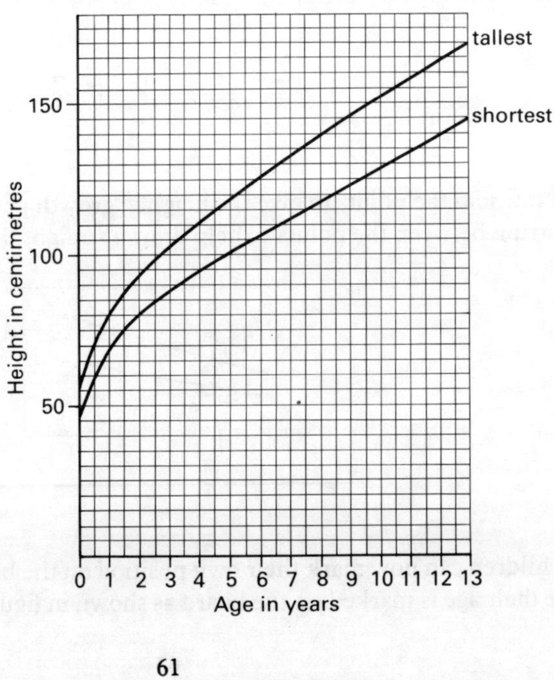

4-16 Age-height chart

greatest and least height at each age. Most children should find that when their height is plotted against their age it will lie between the two lines.

This chart is quite complicated. A simplified chart that covers the ages in primary school can be made because between the ages of 3 and 13 the lines are almost straight.

How to make a simplified chart

(i) Mark an age scale along the bottom of the blackboard (figure 4-17).

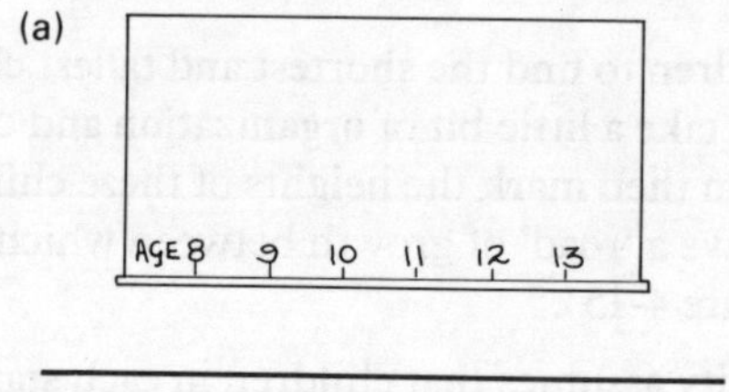

(ii) At the age of 8, the shortest height is 110 cm and the tallest 140 cm. Measure these two distances from the floor and mark them on the board above the age of 8. At the age of 13, the children's heights will lie between 140 cm and 170 cm. Measure and mark these two heights on the board above the age of 13.

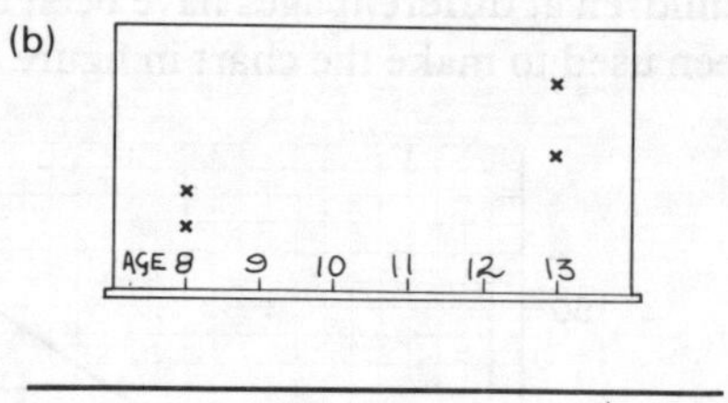

(iii) Now join the points to give the heights' growth path. (Stretch a piece of string between the points to help draw a straight line.)

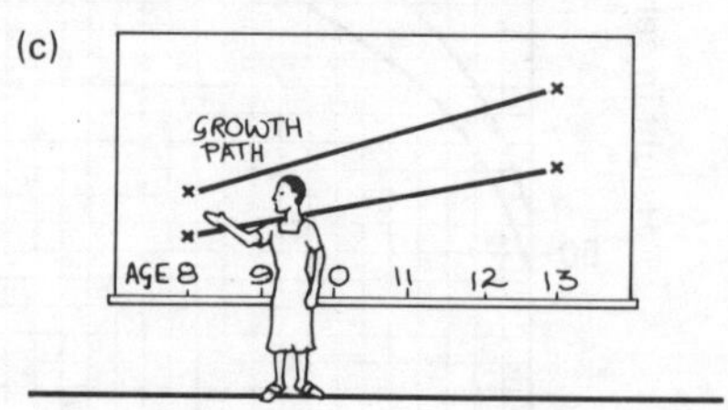

4-17

The children can now mark their own position on the board. Each must stand where their age is marked on the board as shown in figure 4–17 (c).

The children can make a scale drawing of the blackboard chart on squared paper. They can mark their own height and those of their classmates on the chart.

• Activity 12 Upper

• Measuring the height of younger children

The chart drawn in Activity 11 can be used for children between 8 and 13. This chart can now be extended to include younger children.

The children will need to measure the heights of their younger brothers and sisters at home. For each child they can either write down the age and height or cut a stick or piece of string which is the same height as the child. This stick or string can then be marked with the child's name and age and brought to school.

How to draw the standard growth chart for ages 3 to 8

(i) Mark the ages 3 to 8 along the bottom of the board with equal spacing.
(ii) Measure and mark 85 cm and 100 cm from the floor at 3 years. Measure and mark 110 cm and 135 cm from the floor at 8 years.
(iii) Join the marks to make the growth path.

The children can now place their sticks or strings to see if their younger brothers and sisters lie inside the growth path.

The age–height chart is used in some clinics to check that children are growing properly. It is also a good way of introducing children to the concept of the 'road to health'. Children's heights should lie between the two lines on the age–height chart. In the same way children's weights should lie between the lines of the age–weight chart; see Activity 14 in this Chapter.

• Activity 13 Upper

• Predicting adult height

Because the pattern of child growth has been studied in detail it is possible to measure young children and predict the final height to which they will grow.

Children can measure younger brothers and sisters who are two years old (24 months). They can calculate the likely adult height of the child by multiplying their present height by 2.

Example: Jabeta is just 2 years old and is 76 cm tall. The height she is likely to grow to is

$76 \times 2 = 152$ cm or 1.52 m

From the ages of 4 to 9 we can use other multiplying factors (see Table 4-1).

Table 4-1

Age	Multiplying factor Boy	Multiplying factor Girl
4	1.7	1.6
5	1.6	1.5
6	1.5	1.4
7	1.4	1.35
8	1.35	1.3
9	1.3	1.25

The children can use these factors to calculate the future height of younger brothers and sisters.

Example: Salim is 7 years old and 112 cm tall. His adult height is likely to be

$112 \times 1.4 = 156.8$ or 157 cm (to the nearest cm).

So Salim is unlikely to be exactly 157 cm tall but will probably be between 155 cm and 160 cm.

Beyond the age of ten it is not possible to make a reliable prediction.

• Activity 14 — Upper
• The age–weight chart

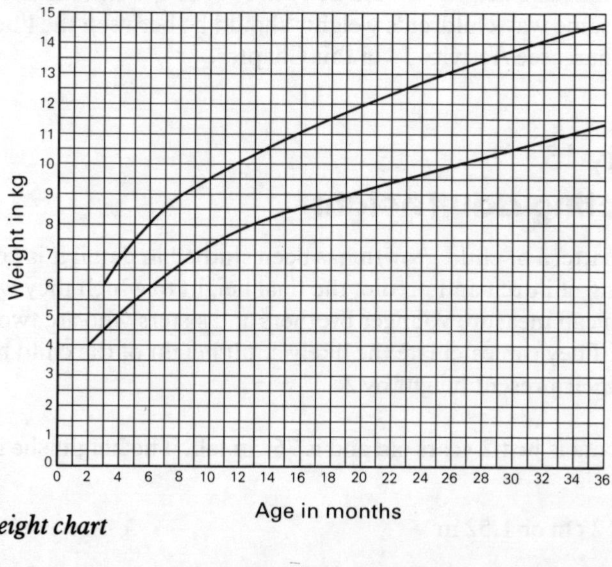

4-18 Age–weight chart

If the children have drawn up a height for age chart using children from their own school, it should now be easier for them to understand the age–weight chart.

The lines showing the tallest and shortest in each standard on the age-height chart are like the two lines on the age–weight chart used in the clinic as shown in figure 4-18.

Most of the children in your class will have weights which lie between these two lines.

If you have a weighing scale then

- show the children how to use the weighing scale then each child can find his or her own weight,
- the children can find the range of weights in the class,
- the children can weigh the lightest and heaviest in each standard and build up a heaviest-lightest chart.

If you do not have a weighing scale then

- set the children the task of finding their own weight,
- arrange with the health clinic for a class visit when young children are being weighed,
- ask the health worker to talk to your class about growth monitoring and the age-weight chart,
- ask the children to bring from home any completed age–weight chart (either their own or that of a younger brother or sister).

Here are Mustapha's weights at different ages (Table 4-2). Use them to plot his growth.

Table 4-2

Age in months	**kg**
3	5
4	5½
5	6
6	6½
7	7
8	7½
9	8

- **Activity 15** **Upper**
- **Interpreting age–weight charts**

Children can learn to interpret the meaning of different dots and lines on the age–weight chart. Here are the charts for three children and some examples of questions that can be asked (figure 4-19).

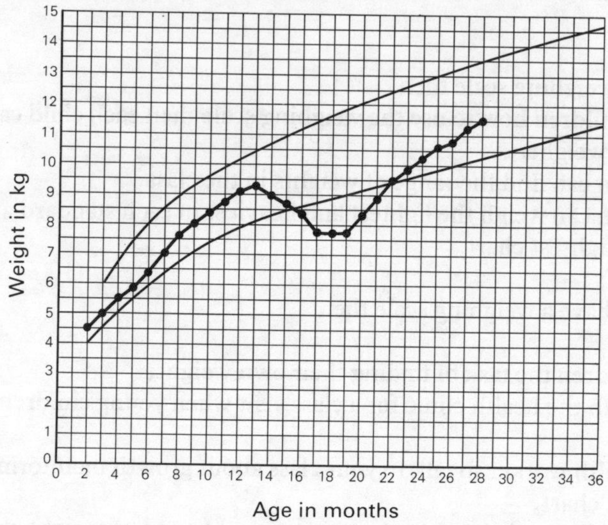

(a) Japhet's chart

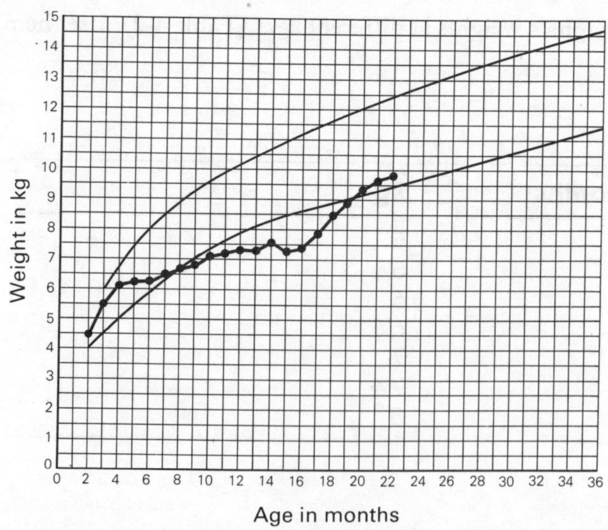

(b) Mbithi's chart

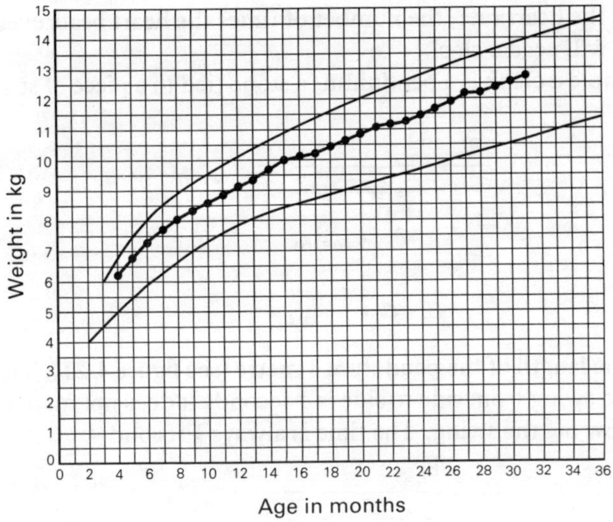

4-19 (c) Mercy's chart

Questions

(1) Which child has grown well?
(2) Which child lost weight after 13 months?
(3) Which child was ill after 4 months?
(4) When did Japhet start to get better?
(5) What weight was Mercy at 2 years?
(6) When did Mbithi start to gain weight fast?
(7) How long did Japhet's illness last?
(8) What do you think Mercy's weight will be by the time she is 3 years old?
(9) Why have the children got different growth charts?

• Activity 16 Upper
• Measuring heart rate

Heart beat is a splendid example of rate. Children can feel their own heart beat by touching the pulse on the wrist. They should put their fingers like this to feel their pulse (figure 4-20).

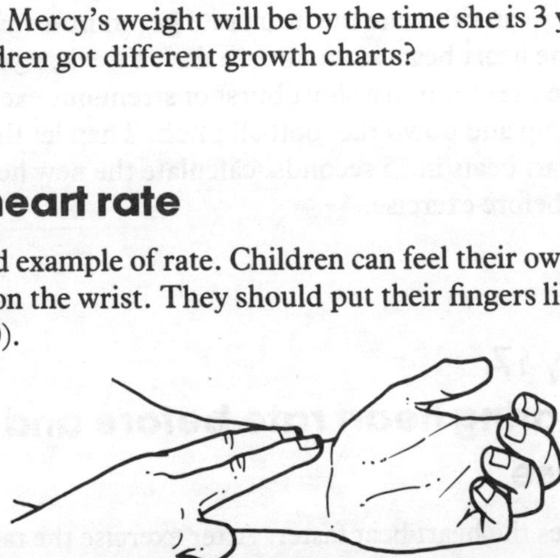

4-20

To find the heart rate, the number of times the heart beats every minute, the children will need a clock.

The simplest clock is a pendulum, a stone tied to a piece of string and swinging.

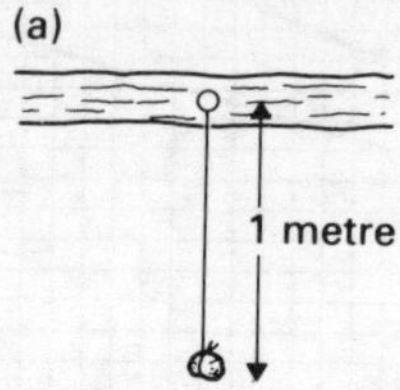

Make the length of the pendulum 1 metre (see figure 4-21). The time the stone takes to swing from side to side is 1 second. It does not matter how big the stone is or how big the swing. The time is always 1 second.

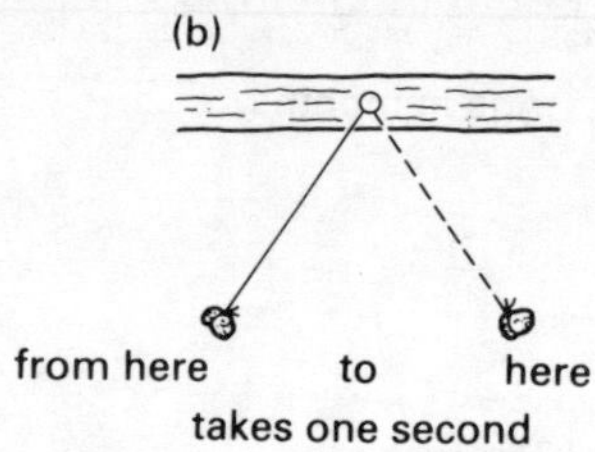

4-21 The simple pendulum

The children can make a metre pendulum and use it to find how many times their pulse beats in 15 seconds. Let the children work in groups with one acting as timekeeper while the others count their pulses.

Then they can calculate the heart rate per minute (and if they like how many times the heart beats in an hour, a day, a week, a year!).

Now give the children a short burst of strenuous exercise: a run around the classroom, or up and down the football pitch. Then let them measure the number of heart beats in 15 seconds, calculate the new heart rate and compare it with the rate before exercise.

• Activity 17 Upper

• Comparing heart rate before and after exercise

Exercise makes the heart beat faster. After exercise the rate gradually falls until it is back to normal. The time it takes for the heart to return to its recovery time is long if you are unfit, short if you are fit.

The children can measure their heart rate after exercise and find how quickly it returns to normal as follows:

(i) the children find their normal heart rate,
(ii) then they take some short sharp exercise,
(iii) then they measure their heart rate every two minutes, counting the pulse beats during 15 seconds (see figure 4-22).

	Pulse beats in 15 seconds	Rate per minute
Before exercise		
After exercise		
After 2 minutes		
After 4 minutes		
After 6 minutes		
After 8 minutes		
After 10 minutes		

4-22

The children can compare results and find

- whose pulse rate returns to normal first,
- whose pulse rate is last to return to normal,
- the ratio of pulse rate before exercise to pulse rate after exercise,
- a way of recording the results for the class on a chart,
- the average pulse rate for the class.

The children can also test older and younger relations at home, making their own pendulum and using it to measure heart rates (see figure 4-23). Here the older child is counting the pulse while his younger sister counts the pendulum swings.

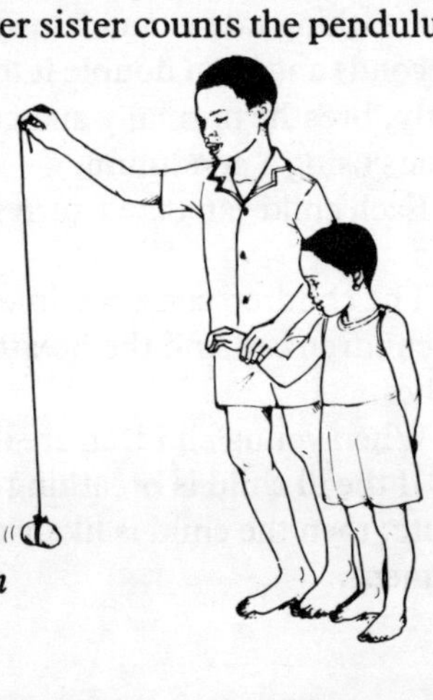

4-23 Measuring heart rate using a simple pendulum

For an adult, 60–80 beats per minute is normal.
For a baby, 100–140 beats per minute is normal.

The chart in figure 4-24 shows the average heart rate at different ages. The children can check against their age and find how their heart rate compares with the average.

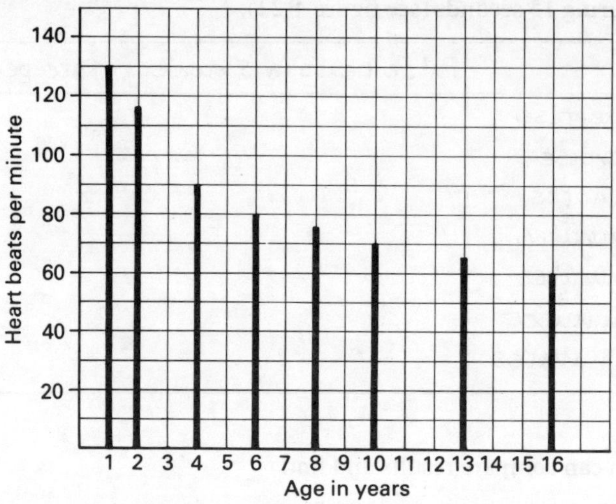

4-24 Average heart rate at different ages

• Activity 18 Upper

• Measuring breathing rate

Breathing rate is more difficult to measure because it is possible to control the rate ourselves.

To measure time use a simple pendulum (see Activity 16 in this Chapter). The breathing rate is much lower than the heart rate. It is best to measure it over 30 seconds and then double it to find the rate per minute. One child can sit quietly, breathe normally and count breaths. A second can measure the 30 seconds using a pendulum.

Each child can take a turn at each activity and record all the results for their group.

The children can experiment to find the effect of exercise on breathing rate. The children can find the breathing rate of younger and older members of their families.

When young children are ill it can be very useful to measure the breathing rate. If the ill child is breathing quickly with a rate of 50 or more breaths per minute, then the child is likely to be suffering from pneumonia and needs treatment.

Exercise

Here are the breathing rates of 4 babies. Which are ill and should be taken to hospital?

Japhet : 18 breaths in 15 seconds
Moli : 15 breaths in 30 seconds
Mary : 17 breaths in 30 seconds
Peter : 26 breaths in 30 seconds

• Activity 19 Upper

• Measuring eyesight

The strength of children's eyesight varies. Some see clearly over a longer distance than others. In this activity the children measure the distance at which they can read a four-figure number.

The children make a set of cards on which are written the four figures 1, 3, 7 and 8. The figures should be about 2 cm high and clearly written.

The children can now work in pairs. One walks a fair distance away while the other arranges the four figure cards to make a number.

The number is held up by one child and the other walks in until he or she can read the number correctly.

The distance from the child to the number is measured and can be called the *eyesight distance*.

Eye sight distance	
1st time	45 m
2nd time	43 m
3rd time	44 m
Average	44 m

4-25

It is a good idea for each child to repeat the activity several times. Each time a new number is used. Each time the eyesight distance is measured. Then the children can calculate the average (see figure 4-25).

The children can calculate the average eyesight distance for the whole class. They can then compare their own eyesight distance with this average.

The children can also investigate whether their two eyes are of equal strength. Each eye is covered in turn and the eyesight distance found for each age.

Measuring eyesight can help you discover which children in your class need to sit at the front or need glasses.

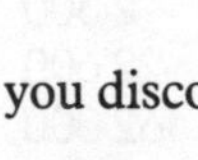

The children can measure the eyesight distance of their younger brothers and sisters. They can identify any children who have eyesight problems.

5 Population

For thousands of years in man's history the level of world population remained remarkably stable. There were slight increases due to periods of peace and plenty and slight decreases due to plagues and wars. But in the present century there has been a dramatic change.

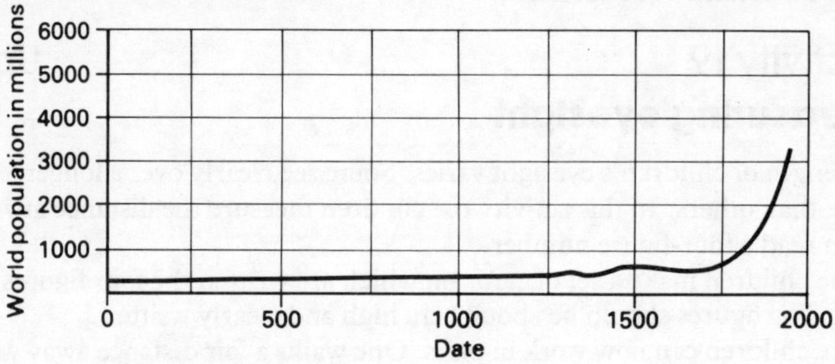

5-1 Chart showing world population

What do you think the world population will be by the year 2000?

Not only has there been a sharp increase in the number of people in the world but also this increase is not evenly shared between the nations. The fastest increase in population is taking place in the developing world. Study the rates of population growth given in Table 5-1.

Table 5-1

	Population in thousands		Birth rate %	Death rate %	Growth rate %
	1985	2000			
Kenya	20 600	38 500	5.5	1.4	4.1
Malawi	6 944	11 400	5.3	2.2	3.1
Tanzania	22 499	39 100	5.0	1.5	3.5
Zimbabwe	6 666	11 200	4.8	1.5	3.3
Zaire	29 938	47 600	4.5	1.6	2.9
Lesotho	1 520	2 300	4.2	1.7	2.5
Ghana	13 588	22 600	4.7	1.5	3.2
Nigeria	95 198	162 000	5.0	1.7	3.3
Uganda	15 477	26 300	5.0	1.7	3.3

Countries with a growth rate of over 3% will double their population in the next 20 years. Find your country in Table 5-1. Has it a growth rate which is greater than 3%?

Table 5-1 gives three different rates, the birth rate, the death rate and the growth rate. These rates are linked closely together:

Growth rate = birth rate − death rate

A SUGGESTED STRATEGY FOR TEACHING ABOUT POPULATION

Population is the study of how many people there are in the world and what kind of people they are. The world is too big and abstract an idea to mean much to the primary school child. Statistics of nations and world population are often so large that they even baffle and puzzle adults.

Can you imagine what this means?

The population of China in 1982 was 1 015 000 000

The strategy for this chapter on population has been to divide the material into four stages.

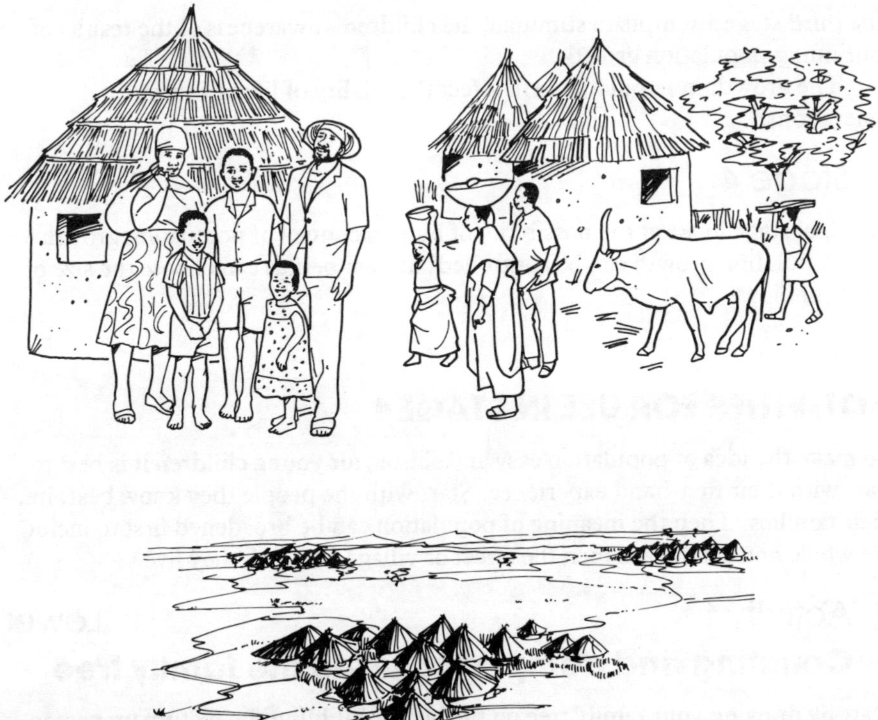

5-2 The home, the village, the district

• Stage 1

The first stage is related most closely to the children's first-hand experience, to facts either about themselves or which they can gather and collect. Then, having collected simple data and learned how to display them in simple forms, the children can compare them to similar charts and graphs made by other children. This helps the children to place their experience in a more universal context.

Each child is part of a family, each family part of a village, each village part of a district, thus each unit goes to make up a larger unit (see figure 5-2).

• Stage 2

The second stage looks at population change by comparing data collected at different times. Now at this stage it is not so easy for the child to collect their own data, so the teaching emphasis shifts from the collection and display of data to the interpretation of charts and graphs.

• Stage 3

The third stage attempts to stimulate the children's awareness of the results of continuing population growth.

The growth in population will affect the quality of life of future generations.

• Stage 4

The final stage looks at the possibility of human control of population growth.

Population growth can be controlled; human beings can choose the size of their families.

ACTIVITIES FOR USE IN STAGE 1

To make the idea of population easy and simple for young children it is best to start with their first-hand experience. Start with the people they know best, i.e. their families. Then the meaning of population can be broadened first to include the whole household and then the street or village in which they live.

• Activity 1 — Lower

• Counting and comparing using the family tree

Start by drawing your family tree on the board, building the picture up person by person. Label the pictures and order the members of the family so that the first born is on the left. Keep the diagram to just those children (living) of your own mother and father (see figure 5-3).

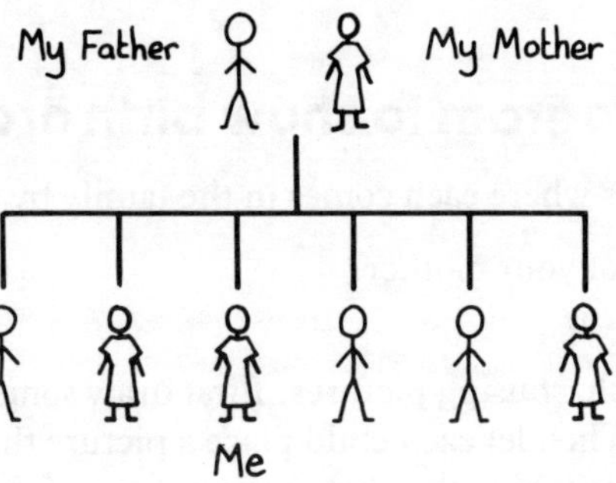

5-3 Illustration of family tree as drawn by the teacher

Ask the children questions about your family tree using as many mathematical ideas as possible. For example,

How many children did my mother have?
Were there more boys than girls?
How many boys?
Where do I come in the family?

Now ask one child to draw their tree on the board following the same pattern as yours. Then ask all the children to make a picture of their own family tree. If you have plenty of paper, this can make an attractive class display.

I have ________ brothers
I have ________ sisters
I am the ________ born
There are ________ males in my family
There are ________ females in my family
I have more ____________ than ____________

5-4

Ask the children questions about their family trees. The children can then write sentences about their own families (see figure 5-4).

• Activity 2 Lower

• Using a pictogram to show birth order

Find out from the class where each comes in the family by asking

Are you the first born of your mother?
Are you the second born?

and so on. Build up a chart using pictures. First draw some rows on the floor or table and label them. Then let each child place a picture they have drawn of themselves in the row to which they belong as in figure 5-5.

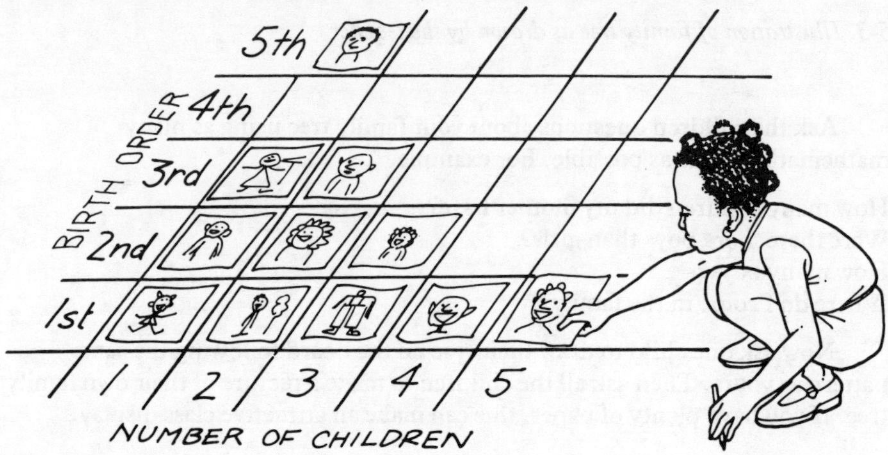

5-5

If you make a copy of the chart on the board, the children can then see how to make their own version on squared paper.

Ask the children questions about their pictogram. For example,

How many children are first born?
Are there more second or third born children in our class?
Which row has most children?

For more ideas on how to make charts and graphs see Chapter 1.

• Activity 3 Middle

• Collecting information, the taller family tree

In Activity 1, children made a simple family tree.

Now extend the idea to include two generations; one pair of grandparents. Once again it will help if you draw your own family tree as an example.

Now ask the children to draw a picture of their own family tree. They will need to gather information from home and this introduces children to the skill of collecting information.

Encourage the children to write mathematical sentences about their tree and to compare it with those of their friends.

• Activity 4 — Middle

• Tabulating information from a household survey

Ask the children in your class to carry out a survey of their household. It will help to prepare with them beforehand a table into which they can put the information they find.

For example, if they collect information on the number of each generation living in their home, then they need a table like the one in figure 5-6 to take home. Each person in the household can then be shown by a single tick.

People with grandchildren							
People with children							
People with no children							

5-6

Alternatively the children can make a survey by age using large or small age intervals. (see figure 5-7).

(a) Age

Over 60 years old								
Over 40 and less than 60								
Over 20 and less than 40								
Under 20 years old								

(b) Age

Over 60						
50 to 59						
40 to 49						
30 to 39						
20 to 29						
10 to 19						
Under 10						

5-7

Choose the survey you think is most suitable for your class situation.

When the children have collected the information you can use it as the basis for a good deal of mathematics. Encourage the children to write short sentences about the data they have found. These can be of the simplest kind:

There are 2 people over 60 in my household.

or it can involve comparison between the data:

There are more people under 10 than over 40 in my household.

Even better, challenge each child to write a set of five questions about their chart for the other children to answer. Make sure they also work out the answers!

Another very valuable exercise which uses the surveys is to pair the children in the class and to ask them to compare their results. Can they make a list of the similarities and the differences?

• Activity 5 — Middle

• Combining household surveys

The data that each child has collected about his or her own household is interesting and valuable, but it may not be typical. A truer picture of the population can be built up by putting together all the children's data. One way to do this is to make a large chart similar to those used by the children in their survey. Let each child add to the chart the information they have collected.

If you feel that there will be too much information if the whole class combines together their data, why not split the class into four groups and let each group make up its own combined chart? You will have four charts about which to ask questions and four charts to compare.

• Activity 6 — Upper

• Understanding national data

Having answered questions about information they have collected themselves, children will find it easier to understand similar data collected by others. Figure 5-8 is an example of a graph made from data collected in the same way as the class data in Activity 5. Here are examples of questions that can be asked on the graph:

How many children are under 10?
How many people are over 60?
How many people are under 20?
How many more people are there between 20 and 30 than between 30 and 40?
Which age-group is the largest?

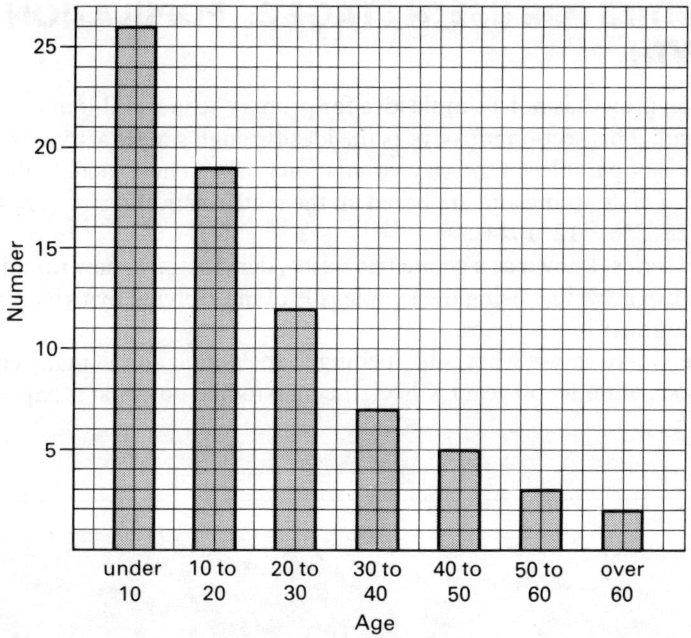

5-8 Chart of population by age in Sanbuku village in 1987

At this stage the simple health message is: there are more children in the world now than ever before. The message becomes even more striking if the children study national data (figure 5-9).

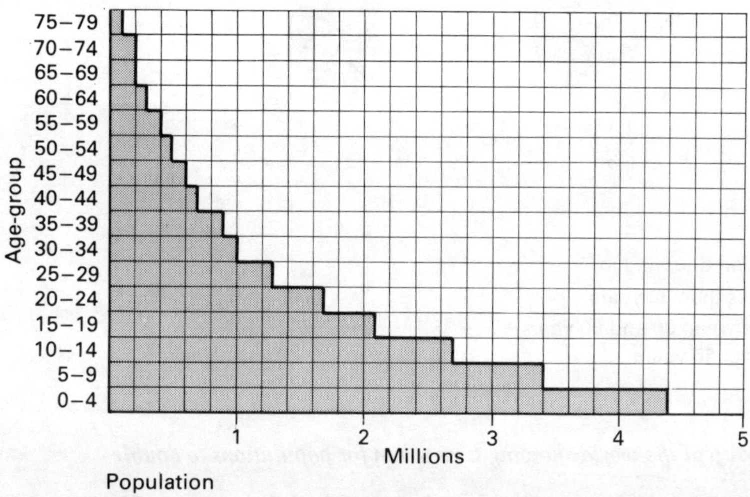

5-9 Population in Kenya by age-group in 1985

ACTIVITIES FOR USE IN STAGE 2: POPULATION GROWTH

Population growth is not a simple idea for primary school children to understand. This section introduces the idea through simple activities which are like models or parables of the way population grows. These models all use the simple idea of doubling and are based on the mathematical series 1, 2, 4, 8, 16, 32, 64, 128, 256, 512, 1024, ...

This series, known as a geometric series, demonstrates how rapidly numbers can grow just using the simple rule of multiplying by two to produce the next number in the series.

Figure 5-10 shows what is happening to the population in many countries over periods of under 30 years. Check the map to find out what is happening in your country.

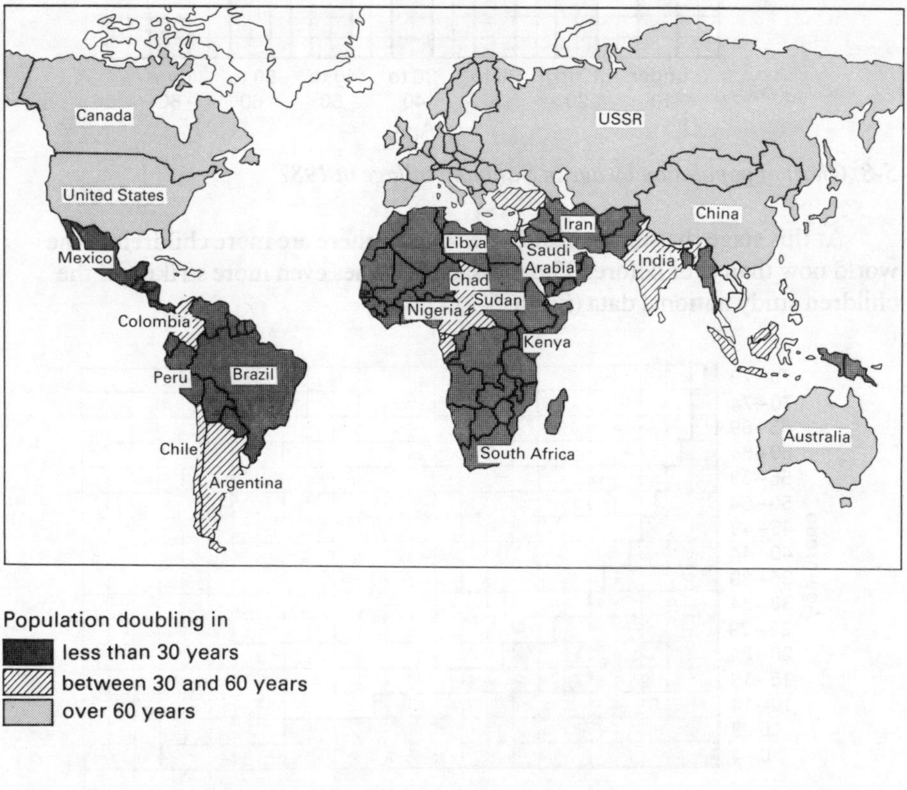

5-10 Map of the world showing time taken for populations to double

So one way of measuring population growth is in terms of how many years it takes for the population to double.

Population growth is also measured as a percentage per year. For example, look at the population figures for a village in Table 5-2. The population has grown by 8. The increase in the population can be given as a percentage.

$$\text{Percentage increase in a year} = \left(\frac{8}{200} \times 100\right)\% = 4\%$$

Table 5-2 Population of village

Year	Population
1987	200
1988	208

All governments keep records of the population collected by national census. These figures can be used to study the growth in population and to calculate the population growth rate in the past. This can then be used to predict (make an intelligent guess at) what is likely to happen in the future.

Doubling time and growth rate are connected

The higher a country's growth rate the shorter will be the time taken for its population to double. A quick approximate way of calculating *doubling time* is to use this mathematical relationship:

$$\text{Doubling time} = \frac{70}{\text{growth rate}}$$

For example, Kenya has a growth rate of about 4%, so

$$\text{Doubling time for Kenya} = \frac{70}{4} \simeq 17 \text{ years}$$

A warning: The percentage growth rate can be used over one year to predict next year's population. When used over more than one year, the problem becomes similar to that of compound interest. Such problems are suitable for investigation with a calculator or in the secondary school but are outside the scope of the standard primary school.

• Activity 7 Middle

• To demonstrate the idea of a doubling population

Mark a circle on the floor or lay down a large loop of string as in figure 5-11. Start with 2 children in the ring. Call this a picture of the year 1940. Tell the children that every 20 years the number in the circle must double. Show them what 1960 looks like. Ask the children how many children will be in the ring in the years (a) 1980 (b) 2000 (c) 2020. See how far you can go with the children before the ring is full.

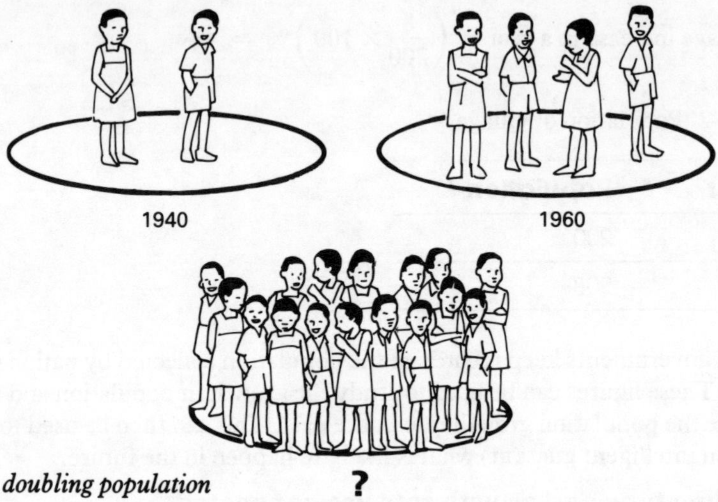

5-11 A doubling population

Here are two other activities which demonstrate the same pattern of growth.

• Activity 8 Middle

• Filling squares with dots to show population doubling

This is an activity that each child can do on squared paper.

Tell the children to put one dot in the first square of a line of squares. Ask them to continue across putting twice as many dots as in the last square in each new square (see figure 5-12). By the time the children reach the 9th or 10th square, the square is almost completely full.

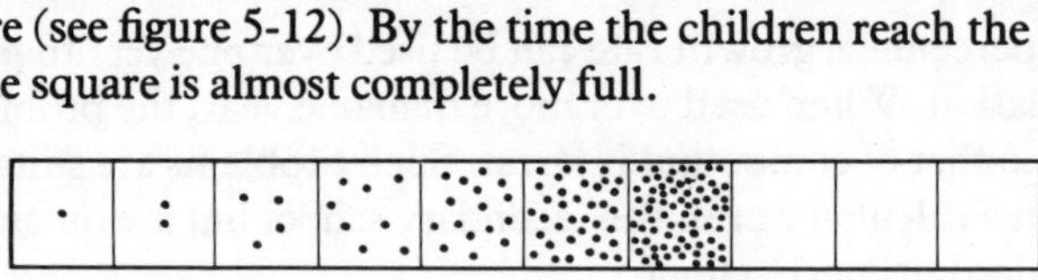

5-12

• Activity 9 Middle

• A doubling population of folded paper people

Folding paper and cutting out paper figures will create the doubling series as well (see figure 5-13).

Newspaper is ideal for this activity and is thin enough to fold up to four times.

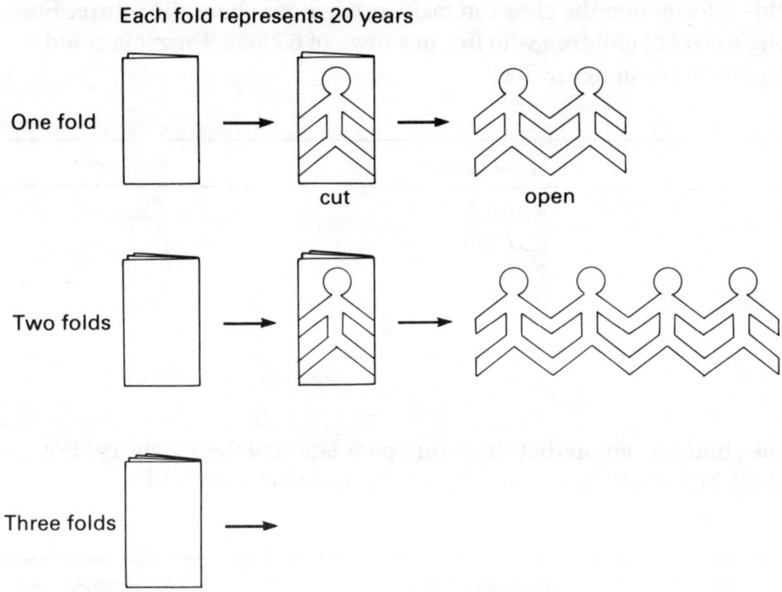

5-13

• Activity 10 — Upper

• Making predictions using doubling times

The last three activities showed simple models of population growth.

In this activity, the children apply the idea of doubling population to their own villages, towns and country.

The children can work out what will happen in the future to their own communities. First they can find from Table 5-3 how many years it takes for their country's population to double.

Table 5-3

Country	Doubling time
Kenya	17 years
Malawi	23 years
Mozambique	25 years
Uganda	21 years
Tanzania	20 years
Zambia	21 years
Zimbabwe	20 years

With this information the class can make predictions about the future. For example, a class of children who live in a town of 6000 in Tanzania could complete the table in figure 5-14.

Year	Population	My age
1990	6,000	?
?	12,000	?
?	?	?
?	?	?

5-14

The children can predict the future population of their country. For example, Kenyan children can complete the table in figure 5-15.

Year	Population	My age
1990	24 million	?
?	?	?
?	?	?
?	?	?

5-15

• Activity 11 Upper

• Using percentage growth rate

Here are some sample mathematical problems based on percentage growth rate.

Calculating growth rate
Here is information about a Kenyan village

Table 5-4

Year	Population
1990	650
1989	625

From Table 5-4 calculate:

(i) the increase in population from 1989 to 1990,
(ii) the percentage population growth from 1989 to 1990.

Using growth rate to predict future population size
The growth rate for a small Tanzanian village is 5% per year.
In 1989 the population was 4000.

(i) Predict the population for 1990.
(ii) Predict the population for 1991.

(These figures have been chosen so it is possible to calculate 5% of the 1990 population.)

Finding growth rate and using it to predict future population
Kambani, a village in Kenya, had a population of 625 in 1987. In 1988 this had grown to 650.

(i) What was the annual percentage growth in the year?
(ii) What do you think the population might be in 1989?

ACTIVITIES FOR USE IN STAGE 3: THE CONSEQUENCES OF POPULATION GROWTH

Population growth is a threat to development because of the increasing burdens it places on a nation's resources. An increasing population means, for example, an increasing demand for

- land
- housing
- schools
- food
- jobs

A striking illustration of the way the efforts of a country can be used up by just providing for the new population is shown by these statistics from India.

Simply to stand still in the services it provides, India needs

- 190 million extra metres of cloth
- 10 million extra tonnes of food
- 127 000 extra schools
- 4 million extra jobs
- 373 000 extra teachers

How many babies are born in Kenya every year? In Kenya the population is about 20 million. The birth rate is 5% per year. What will they need as they grow up?

The problem of sharing and inheriting land is familiar to many communities. Where the farm or shamba has to be shared equally between all the sons then the result after each generation is smaller and smaller plots of land. The first activity in this section attempts to model this problem.

• Activity 12 **Middle**

• Sharing out land

Each child should draw an 8 by 8 square on squared paper (figure 5-16). This is a map of their land. Each small square represents 1 hectare. Let them find the area of their land (64 hectares). Tell the class: 'You have two children. Divide the land (show it on your map) so that each child has an equal share. How much land has each child?'

(a)

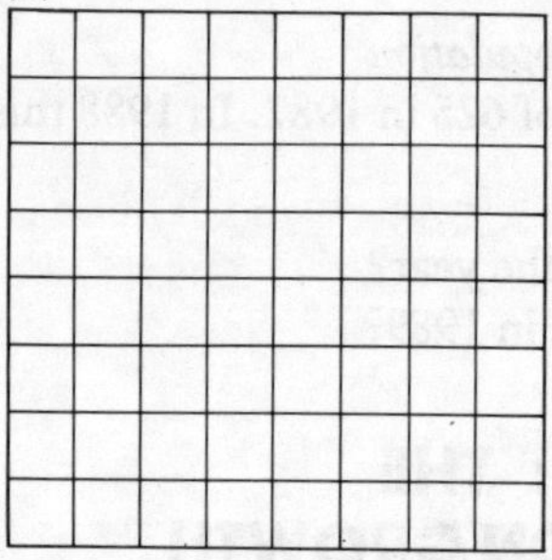

(b)

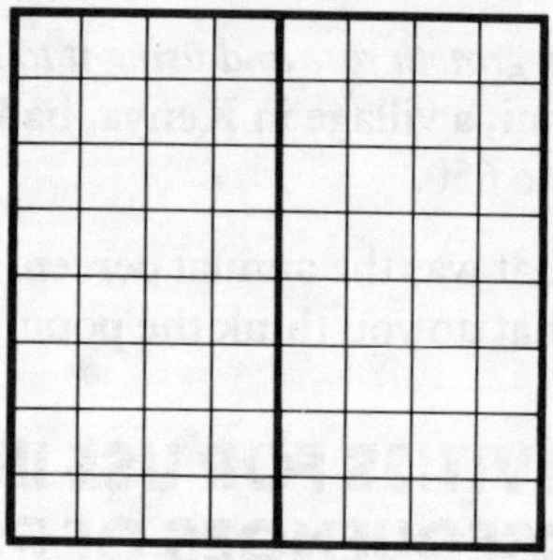

Continue the story through several generations: 'Each child has two children i.e. you have four grandchildren. Divide the land for them.'

(c)

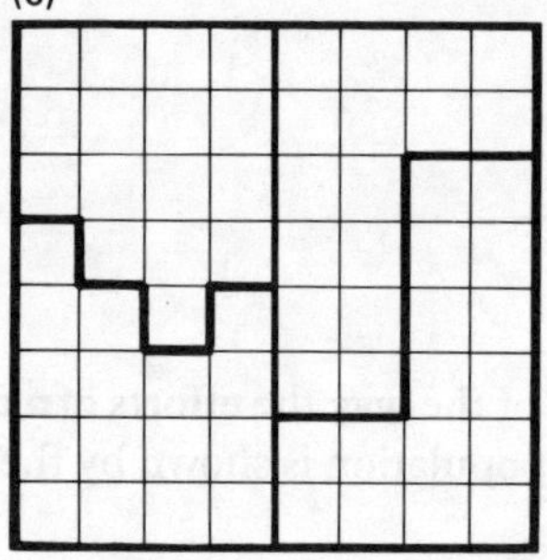

At each generation, get the children to draw the new divisions and write down how much land a child has got. How many generations will it be before each child has only 1 hectare of land?

(d)

Generation	Land(hectares)
1	64
2	32
3	16
4	8
5	4
6	2
7	1

5-16

Further activity

Starting each time with an 8 by 8 square, let each child in the class investigate what happens if:

(a) they have 4 children and each of these children has 4 children, and so on,
(b) they have 8 children and each of these children has 8 children.

• Activity 13 Middle/upper

• Calculating land available for farming

Each child draws their own outline on squared paper. The outline should contain 64 squares but can be any shape they like. Each square represents 100 m^2 in this activity and the outline represents a piece of land. Then ask each child to 'build' two houses on the land, each house to be shown by shading a square. The land can then be divided equally between the houses. The children then calculate how much land each household has for farming:

Households = 2
Land for farming (64 − 2 = 62) = 6200 m^2
Each household has 6200 ÷ 2 = 3100 m^2

Ask the children to find out what happens as the population continues to double. How soon will there be no land left?

• Activity 14 Middle/upper

• Representing population on a map

Draw a simplified map of Uganda, Kenya and Tanzania on your squared board (see Appendix). Using a scale of 🯅 equals 1 million people, let the children fill in the data for 1920 (figure 5–17 (a)):

Uganda = 4 million
Kenya = 4 million
Tanzania = 5 million

(a)

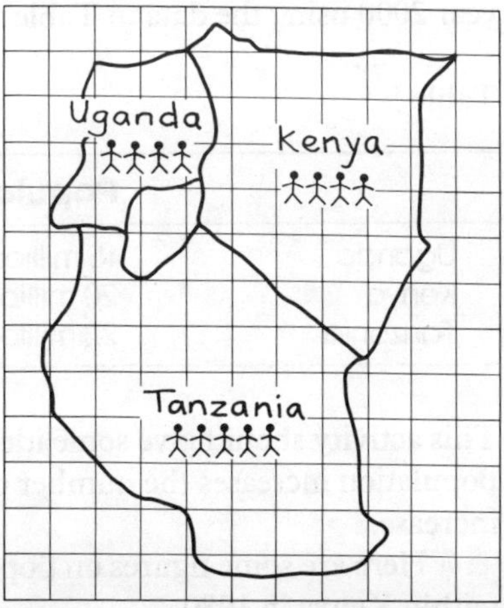

5-17 (a) Population in Uganda, Kenya and Tanzania in 1920

Now let the children fill in on another map the information for 1960 (figure 5-17 (b)):

Uganda = 8 million
Kenya = 10 million
Tanzania = 12 million

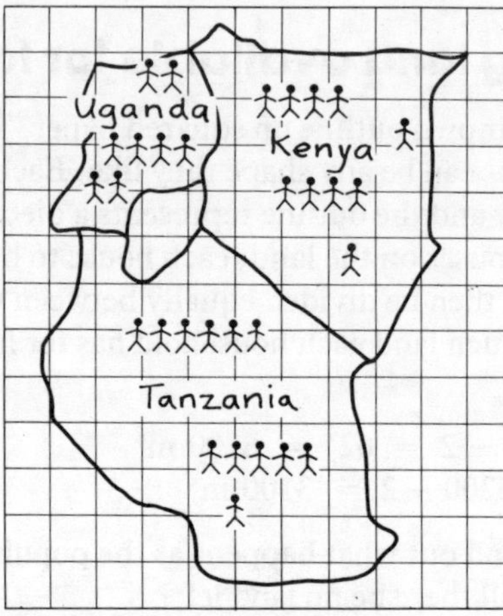

5-17 (b) Population in Uganda, Kenya and Tanzania in 1960

For the next activity it might be a good idea to let each child make two copies of the map (if they draw on squared paper they will find it easier to copy your map). Then the children can use their maps to draw pictograms for 1985 and the year 2000 using the data in Table 5-5 to fill in the correct number of stick men.

Table 5-5

	Population in 1985	Population in 2000
Uganda	15 million	26 million
Kenya	20 million	39 million
Tanzania	22 million	39 million

This activity should give some idea of the growing density of population. As the population increases the number of people per square kilometre will also increase.

Here are some figures on population density (Table 5-6) in some provinces within Kenya in 1980:

Table 5-6

Provinces	Population density (people/km²)
Central	250
Coast	100
Eastern	100
Nyanza	200
Rift Valley	100
Western	250

Suggested exercise
Calculate the average amount of land for each person in each province. For example,

In Central province there are 250 people for every 1 km^2
1 km^2 = 100 hectares
So there are 250 people per 100 hectares

or 1 person per $\frac{100}{250} = 0.4$ hectare

Supplementary exercise
In the year 2000 the population will be twice that in 1980. Work out what you think will be the average amount of land per person for each province in that year.

ACTIVITIES FOR USE IN STAGE 4: POPULATION CAN BE CONTROLLED

The topic of birth control does not lie within the scope of this book. Here instead are a few ideas that may help to raise the pupils' awareness of family size and family spacing.

(a)

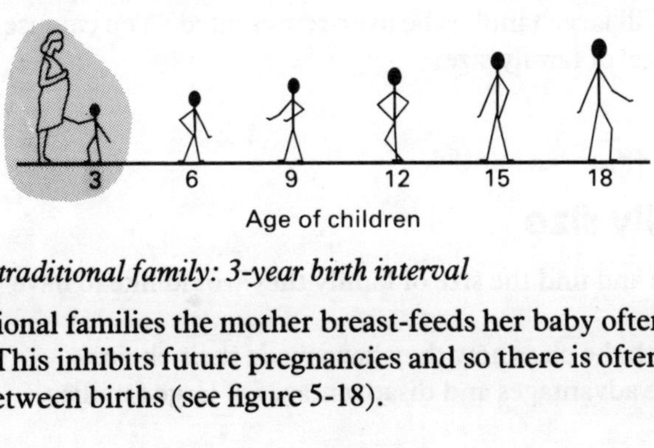

5-18 (a) The traditional family: 3-year birth interval

In traditional families the mother breast-feeds her baby often and over a long period. This inhibits future pregnancies and so there is often an interval of three years between births (see figure 5-18).

With modern families the picture is different

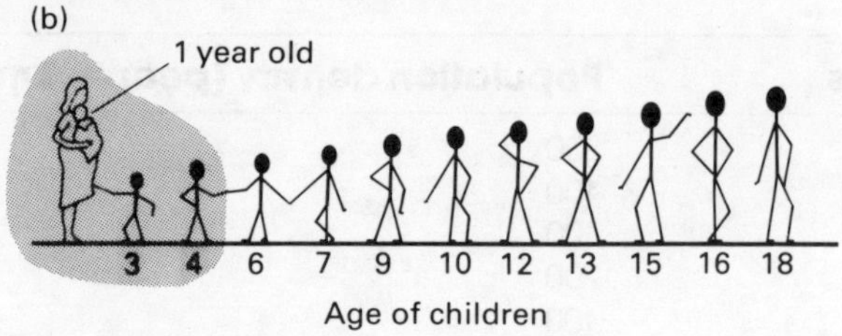

5-18 (b) The modern family: $1\frac{1}{2}$-year birth interval

In the modern family there are more children, more closely spaced. The effects of this are that the children and the mother suffer both mentally and physically.

The results of longer birth intervals are

- lower health risks for mother and baby,
- taller and heavier children,
- more attention given to young children by mothers,
- brighter and more intelligent children.

Through the activities in Stage 4, children can be made aware of the range of family size that already exists within their own community. They can also learn that children can be spaced at different intervals so that in some families the children come close together in age, in other families their ages are more widely spaced.

• Activity 15 — Upper

• The range of family size

Survey the class to find the size of the family to which each child belongs. It helps if the 'family size' is defined as the 'number of children from your mother'.

You can discuss with the children whether this gives a true picture of 'families' in the community. Will a husband and wife with no children be shown on this chart? Will large families be over-represented? You can use the survey to discuss the 'range' of family size.

• Activity 16 — Upper

• My family size

Survey the class and find the size of family they would like to have when they become parents.

Discuss with the class how they have made their choice.

Discuss the advantages and disadvantages of large families.

• Activity 17 Upper

• Family size and predicting future population

In Activity 16 the children chose the number of children they would like. In this activity they study the effect family size will have on population. At present in Kenya the average family size, or number of children per mother, is 8. If 8 children remains the average, then the predicted growth of population is shown in figure 5–19 (a). The dark section of the graph shows the population under 15 years old.

(a)

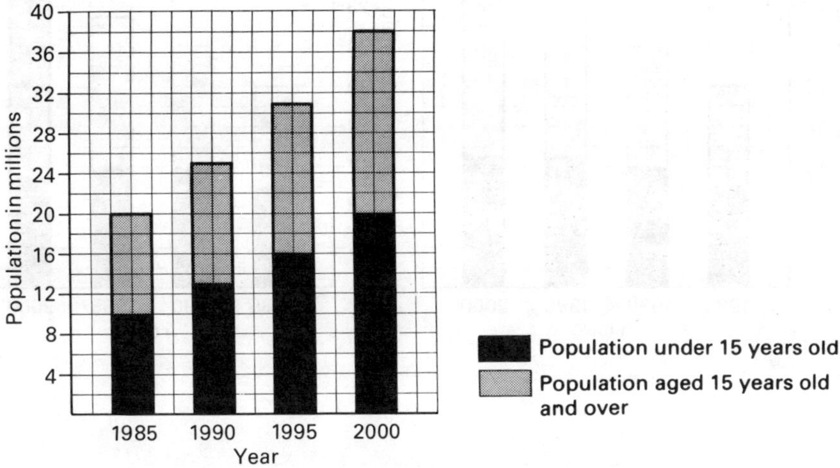

If the average number of children falls to 6, then the population will not grow so rapidly. Figure 5-19 (b) shows the population predicted.

(b)

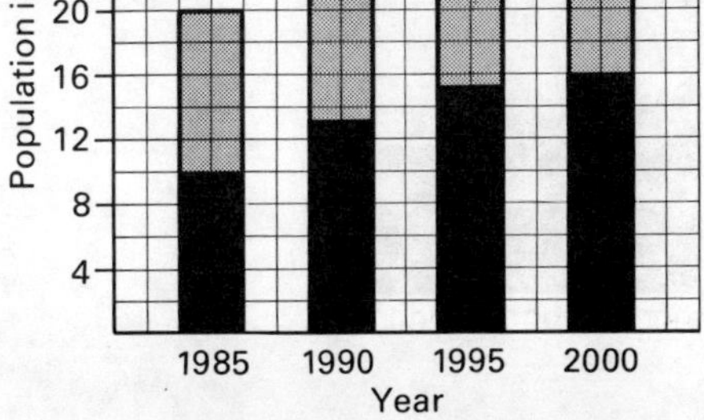

5-19 Predicted growth of population in Kenya for family with (a) 8 children per mother (b) 6 children per mother

The children can study the graphs in figure 5-20 and see what will be the result of their choice of family size.

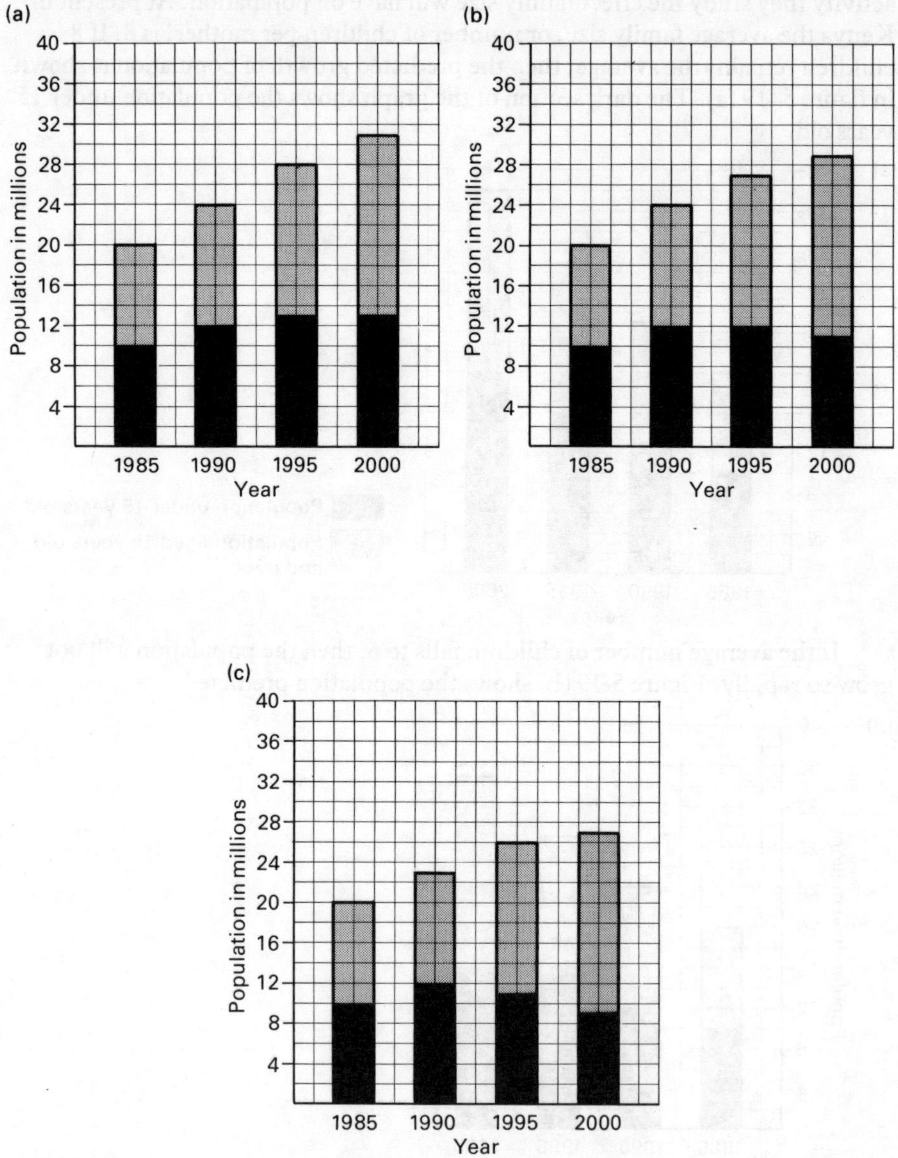

5-20 Predicted growth of population in Kenya for family with (a) 4 children per mother (b) 3 children per mother (c) 2 children per mother

Here are some possible exercises that can be set on the graphs.

(1) Find the increase in population over 15 years from 1985 to 2000 for each graph.
(2) Study the population of children under 15. Does it increase in each graph?
(3) How many more children under 15 will there be in the year 2000 than in 1990 if the family size remains at 3 children per mother?

• Activity 18 Upper
• Using a time line to show birth interval

Investigate the birth interval between children. Figure 5-21 is an example of a time line showing when each child in a family was born.

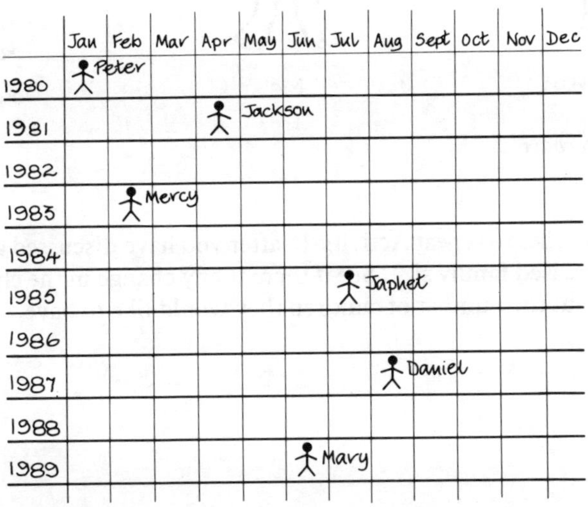

5-21

The birth intervals can be found from the chart.

The birth interval between Peter and Jackson is 15 months.
The birth interval between Jackson and Mercy is 22 months.

Each child can make a birth interval chart and calculate the average birth interval for their family. Then the class average can be found.

For a simpler exercise, just ask for the birth intervals for the brothers and sisters born before and after the children in your class (figure 5-22). You can use the children's data as a starting point for discussing the advantages of increased birth intervals.

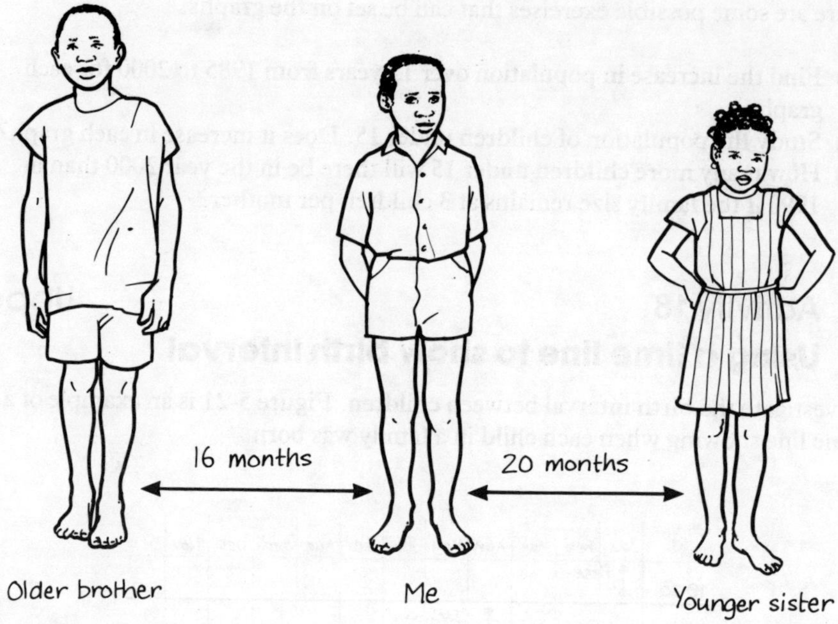

5-22 Birth intervals

You might like to repeat Activity 16 after you have discussed all the issues relating to increased family size. See if there is any change in the choices the class make about the number of children they would like to have.

6 Nutrition and breast feeding

(a)

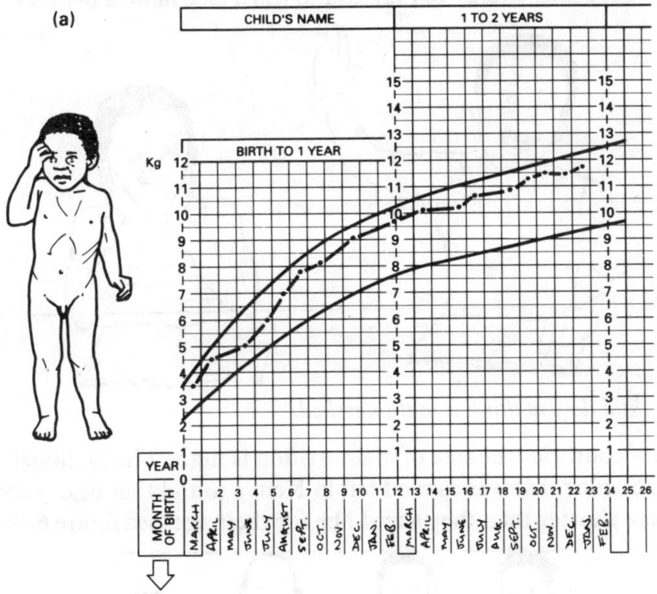

(b)

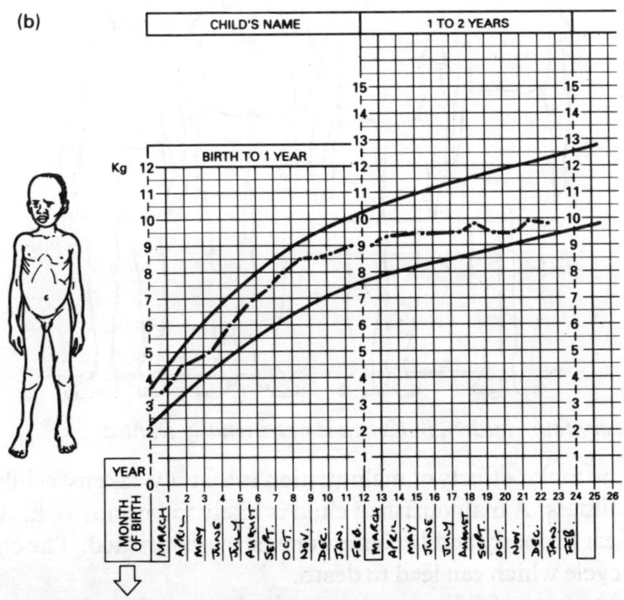

6-1 (a) Growth chart for child showing good growth (b) Growth chart for child showing poor growth

For good growth children need to eat the right amount of food and the right kind of food. Without it children suffer from malnutrition, their growth is stunted and they lack energy to play and to learn (see figures 6-1 and 6-2).

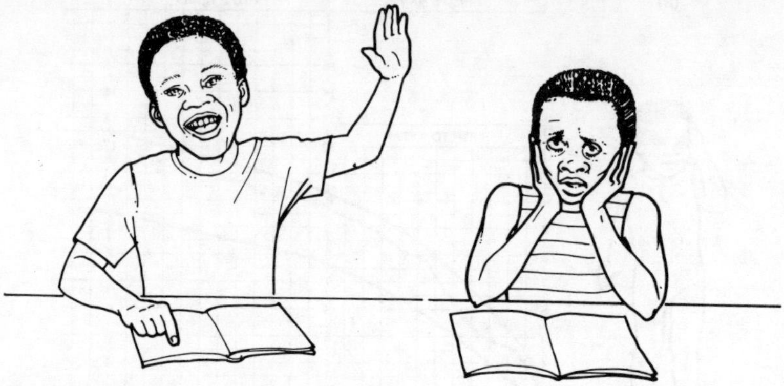

6-2 Which child do you think is malnourished?

In many countries the rate of malnutrition is high. The National Nutritional Survey that was carried out in Kenya found that nearly 25% of all children were shorter than they should be for their age (see figure 6-3).

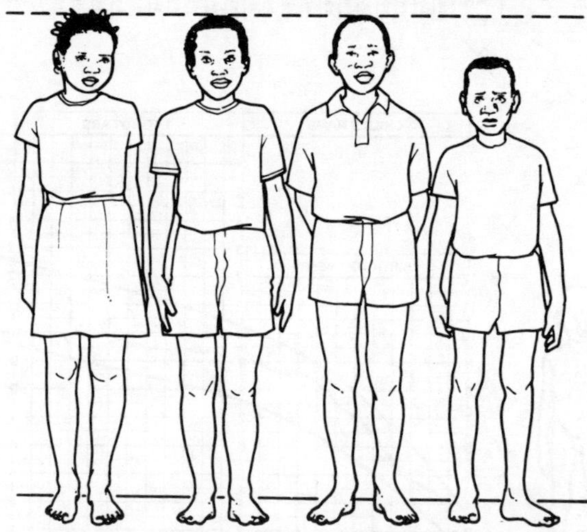

6-3 One in every four children in Kenya is nutritionally stunted

One of the major effects of malnutrition is that it weakens a child's resistance to illness. A malnourished child is likely to become sick. A sick child often fails to eat properly and becomes further malnourished. The child is trapped in a cycle which can lead to death.

The effect of poor feeding can be seen in the rate of deaths among young children. This infant death rate varies from country to country and area to area (see figure 6-4). What is the infant death rate in your country?

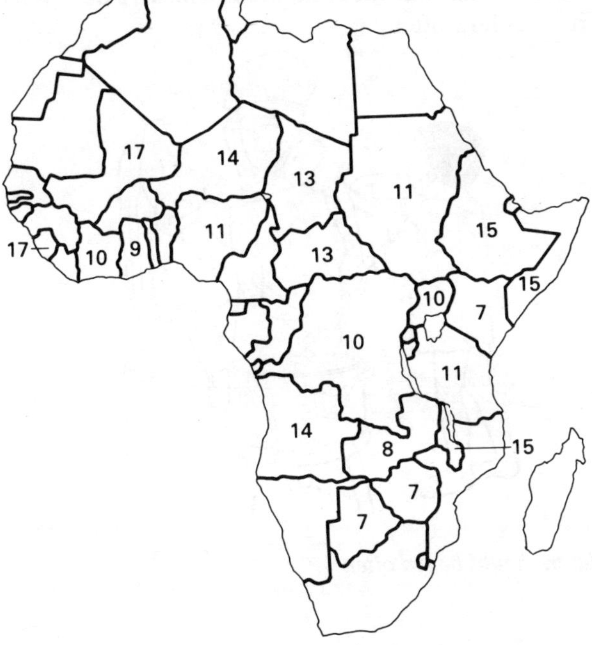

6-4 Percentage of children dying in Africa before the age of one

Malnutrition contributes to these high death rates. It also leaves many millions more children who survive and grow to be adults but whose intellectual and physical growth has been damaged and stunted.

Proper feeding of children will prevent malnutrition. For the young baby from birth to the age of 4 to 6 months, the mother's milk provides the best possible diet. It contains all that the body needs to grow and helps protect the baby against illness. At this age the baby needs to be fed as often as the baby wishes.

Between 4 and 6 months after birth, the baby starts to need extra food. The mother's milk alone is not enough to make the baby grow well and other foods need to be given as well as breast milk. These extra foods should be:

- high in energy: fat, oil or sugar mixed with staple foods and fruits,
- easy to digest,
- pure and clean,
- given in little amounts and often.

From the age of 2 years until the child is 5 years old, the child needs at least 5 meals a day. From 5 years on, the child needs 3 meals a day. What the child eats is as important as how often.

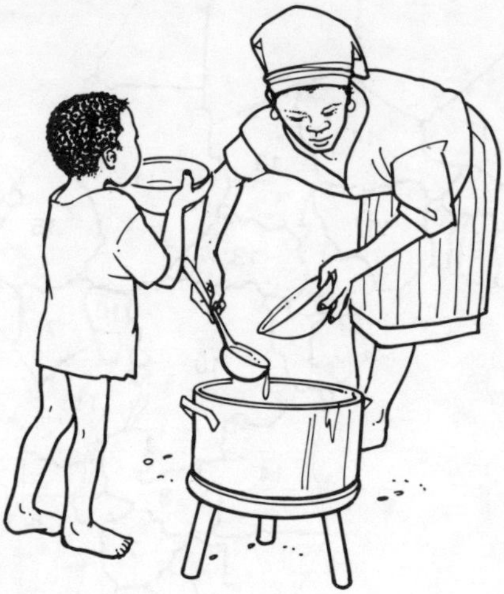

6-5 Young children should be fed often

To help the body develop, the child needs food for growth (**Grow foods**)

Beans	Chicken	Eggs
Milk	Meat	Fish
Ground nuts	Flying ants	Caterpillars

The child needs foods that give energy (**Go foods**)

Cooking oil	Bread	Maize porridge
Sugar	Rice	Bananas
Potatoes	Margarine	Millet
Sugar cane	Nuts	

The child needs foods that give protection against disease (**Glow foods**)

Pumpkin	Pineapple	Paw paw	Guavas
Green leaves	Lemon	Mango	Pepper
Tomatoes	Onions	Orange	Peas
Cabbage			

Here are some activities that link some of these ideas about nutrition to mathematics.

• Activity 1 Middle

• Meal survey

The number of meals children eat is a rough guide to whether or not they are getting sufficient food. It is especially important that young children eat often.

The children can carry out a class survey to find how many meals each child in the class ate yesterday.

The children can display the results in the form of a chart like the one in figure 6-6.

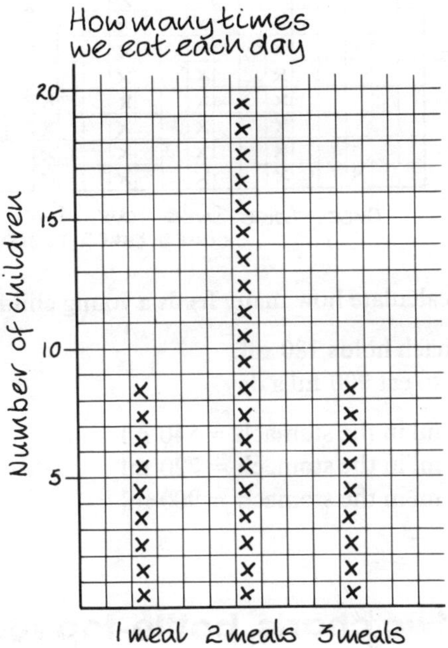

6-6

Discuss with the children the value of frequent meals. Children should eat often (see figure 6-7).

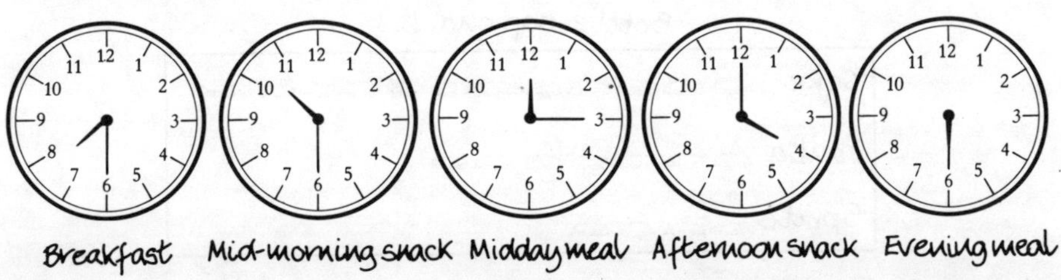
Breakfast
Mid-morning snack
Midday meal
Afternoon snack
Evening meal

6-7

The children can now carry out a survey of their own homes. They can find out how often the children under 2 years old feed each day.

Figure 6-8 shows a table of what the results might look like. Ask the children to identify the children who are not having enough feeds every day.

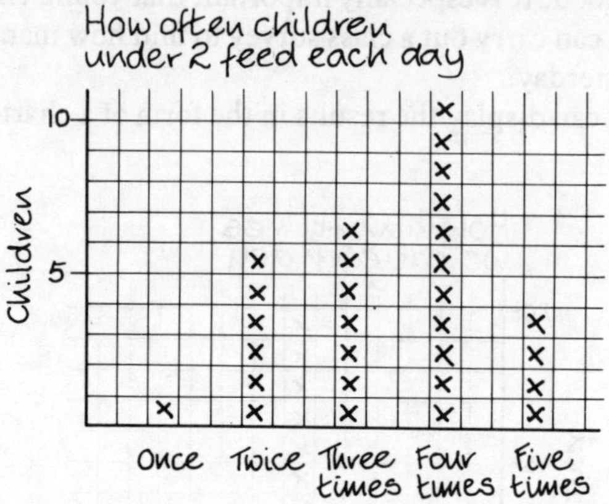

6-8

The children can now calculate how many feeds a young child needs.

The young child's stomach holds 180 ml.
The young child needs to eat 900 ml a day.

3 meals a day: 3 × 180 ml in the stomach = 540 ml
4 meals a day: 4 × 180 ml in the stomach = 720 ml
5 meals a day: 5 × 180 ml in the stomach = 900 ml

• Activity 2 Middle

• Comparing two charts, bottle-top survey

Get the children to collect all the bottle-tops they can find that come from soft drinks.

Let them build a bottle-top chart to show the popularity of each drink, like the one in figure 6-9.

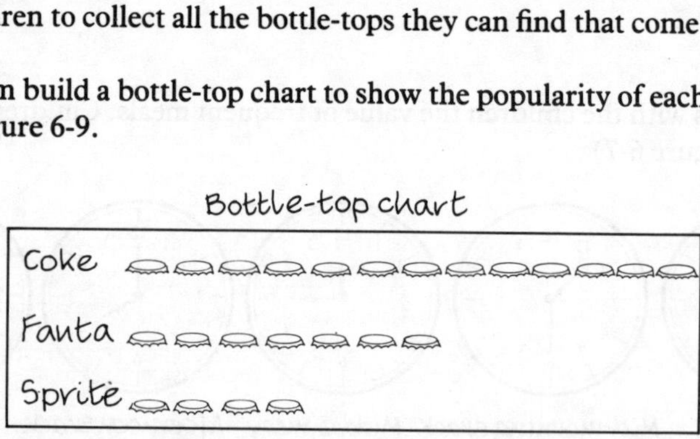

6-9 Chart showing bottle-tops laid out in lines according to type

The children can then carry out a class survey to find out each child's favourite drink (see figure 6-10).

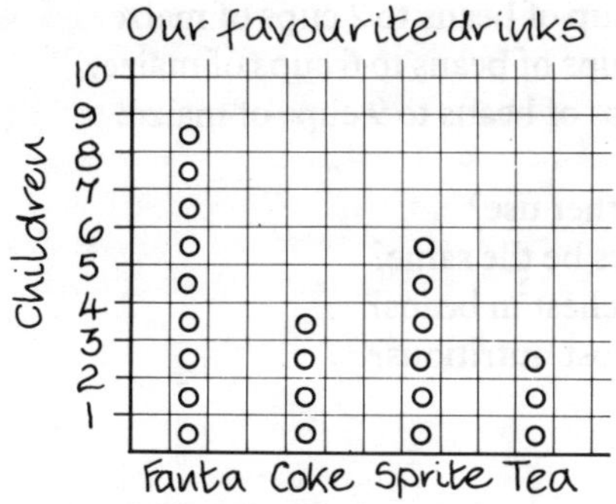

6-10 Class survey of our favourite drinks

The children can compare the two charts.

Questions

Here are some questions that the children can answer based on the charts in figures 6-9 and 6-10.

(1) Which was the most popular drink according to the bottle-top graph in figure 6-9?
(2) Which was your class favourite?
(3) How many bottles must there have been to give all the bottle-tops?
(4) How much had been spent to buy all these bottles of drink?
(5) How many oranges could be bought for the price of a bottle of Coke?
(6) Which is more nutritious, an orange or a Coke?

• Activity 3 — Middle

• Understanding ratios, mixing food

When food is mixed in the preparation of meals, the different kinds of food are added in a given ratio.

For example, when maize porridge is made, maize flour and water are mixed. If 1 cup of maize flour is added to 4 cups of water, then the ratio of maize flour to water is 1 : 4. The children can find out what ratio their mother uses at home and compare ratios. The children can also use their ratios to find how much water must be added to 2 cups, 3 cups or 5 cups of maize flour.

The children can investigate the ratios used in mixing other foods, for example, beans and maize. The children can compare the ratios used in different homes and decide which mixtures are richer in beans and so more nutritious.

For example,

Martha's mother uses 1 cup of beans to 2 cups of maize.
Joseph's mother uses 2 cups of beans to 6 cups of maize.
Peter's mother uses 3 cups of beans to 9 cups of maize.

What ratio does each mother use?
Will any of these mixtures be the same?
Which mixture will be richest in beans?
Which mixture will be most nutritious?

• Activity 4 — Middle

• Feeding survey of young children

Children are most likely to become malnourished between the ages of 6 months and 1 year. For the first 4 months, children should be breast fed. From 4 months, they should have other nutritious foods as well.

The children can carry out a survey on babies under 1 year old in their households and find how they are being fed. A sample question sheet is shown in figure 6-11.

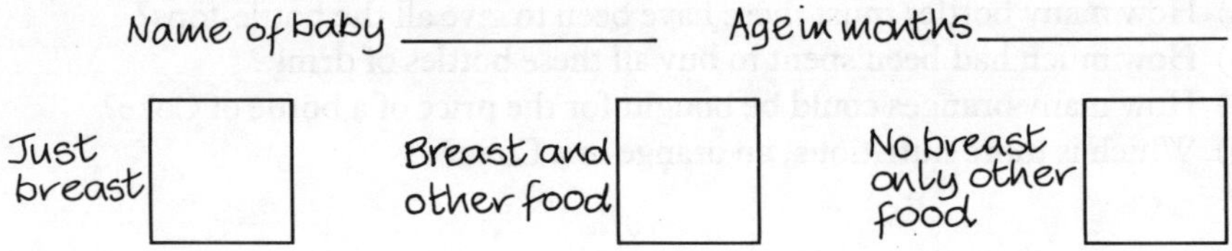

6-11

The children tick just one box. One way to display all the answers collected by the class is for the children to make three charts. Each baby is entered on to just one of these charts. The children can answer questions on the charts.

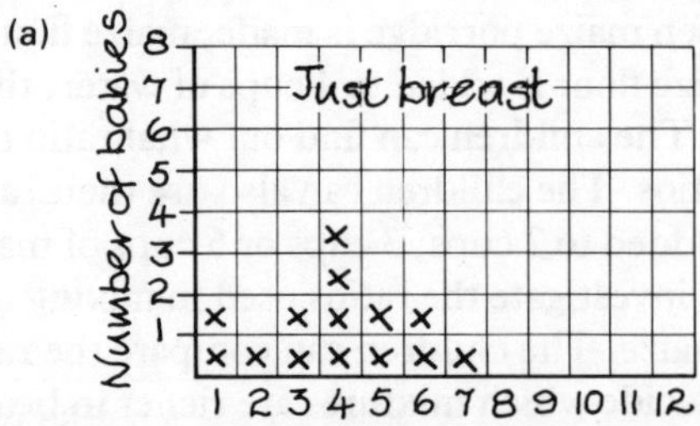

Figure 6-12(a) shows a chart for the babies fed just breast milk. How many babies over 4 months are still being breast fed? Which children need other food as well as breast milk?

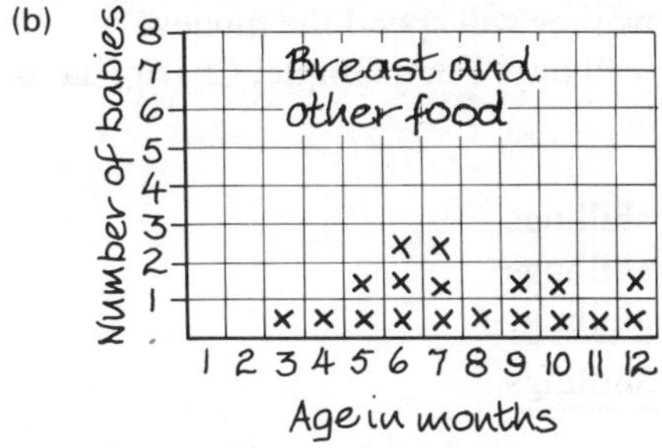

Figure 6-12(b) shows a chart for those babies fed breast milk and other food. How many babies under 5 months are being fed other food?

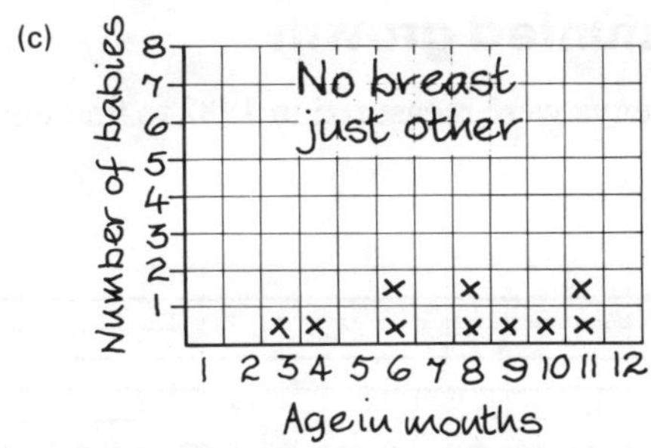

6-12 Charts for babies fed (a) just breast milk (b) breast milk and other food (c) no breast milk, just other food

Figure 6-12(c) shows a chart for those babies fed no breast milk, just other food. How many children are not being fed breast milk? Are these children being fed properly?

• Activity 5 Middle

• Problem solving, buying a balanced meal

There are three types of food the body needs for a balanced diet. Examples are given on page 98.

Draw three market stalls; one will have energy foods, one will have growth foods, and the third will have protection foods.

The children can suggest which foods go on each stall. They can also decide on the price of each.

Let the children imagine that they have a certain amount of money to spend on food. They must buy food from each stall so that they have a balanced meal. Each child can decide how they will spend the money.

They list what they will buy. For example, Charity has 6 shillings and decides to buy

2 bananas (energy)	2 shillings
1 egg (growth)	2 shillings
1 cabbage (protection)	2 shillings
Total	6 shillings

The children can investigate all the different ways in which Charity's money can be spent to buy a balanced meal.

• Activity 6 Upper

• Statistics of stunted growth

Children throughout Kenya were measured in 1982 to find out if they were growing properly.

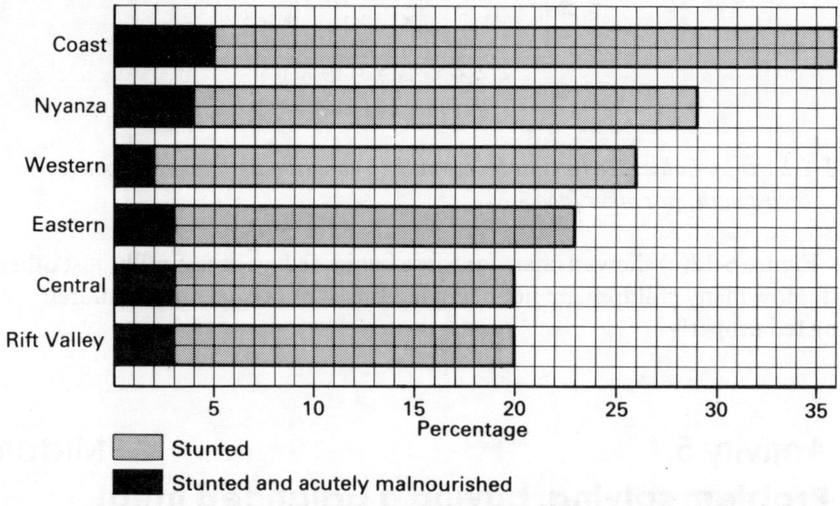

6-13 Percentage of under fives with stunted growth in Kenya in 1982

Figure 6-13 shows the results. 'Stunted growth' means the children have not reached their proper height due to long-term undernutrition.

The children can use the graph to find the percentage of stunted children in each province.

They can also use the percentage to find how many children under 5 in each province are likely to be malnourished. Here are the under-5 populations for each province in Kenya.

Coast	440 000
Nyanza	920 000
Western	640 000
Central	780 000
Rift Valley	1 180 000
Eastern	920 000

Find the number of stunted children in Western province from figure 6–13:

From the graph, 26% are stunted in Western province.

$$\text{The number of children stunted} = \frac{26}{100} \times 640\ 000$$

$$= 166\ 400$$

To find the number of children suffering from acute malnutrition in Nyanza province:

From the graph, 4% are acutely malnourished in Nyanza province.

$$\text{The number of children acutely malnourished} = \frac{4}{100} \times 920\ 000$$

$$= 36\ 800$$

The children can complete similar calculations for other provinces.

• Activity 7 Upper

• Understanding a chart about breast feeding

No milk substitute has ever been invented which so perfectly meets the needs of a growing baby as mother's milk. Mother's milk also helps to protect babies when they are most at risk from disease in the first months of life.

The chart in figure 6-14 shows the number of deaths among babies. The babies were fed in three different ways.

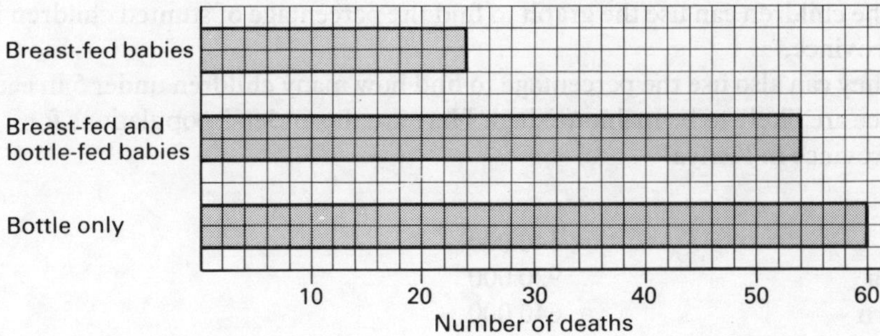

6-14 Deaths among 1000 babies

Sample questions on the chart

(1) How many bottle-fed babies died?
(2) How many breast-fed babies died?
(3) How many more bottle-fed babies died than breast-fed babies?
(4) Why do you think there is this difference?
(5) How would you like your baby to be fed?

• Activity 8 Upper

• Using a weight-for-age table

Table 6-1 shows the weight below which a child of a given age is malnourished.

For example, a child of 7 months has a weight of 5.8 kg. From the table it can be seen that a child of 7 months should not weigh less than 6 kg, so this child is malnourished.

Table 6-1

Age of child in months	**Weight below which child is malnourished (kg)**
2	3.4
3	4.0
4	4.6
5	5.1
6	5.6
7	6.0
8	6.4
9	6.7
10	7.0
11	7.3
12	7.6

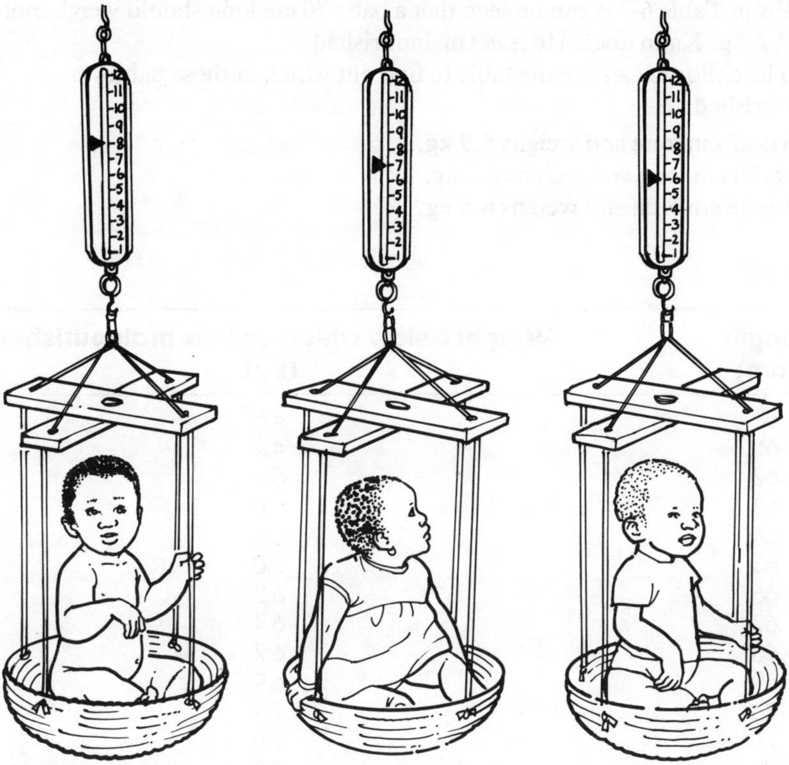

Mubita 11 months Kakoma 8 months Mondia 10 months

6-15

Exercise using Table 6-1
The children can find the weight of each baby in figure 6-15 by reading the scale.

Then the children can use Table 6-1 to check whether or not each baby is malnourished.

• Activity 9 Upper
• Using a height–weight table

Table 6-2 shows the weight a child should have for a given height or length and the weight below which the child would be malnourished.

Here is a sample exercise based on the table. Kalin is 70 cm long. He weighs 8.2 kg. Is he malnourished?

From Table 6-2 it can be seen that a baby 70 cm long should weigh more than 7.2 kg. Kalin does. He is *not* malnourished.

The children can use the table to find out which of these babies is malnourished:

Jacob is 67 cm long and weighs 6.9 kg.
Ruth is 78 cm long and weighs 8.7 kg.
Salim is 63 cm long and weighs 6.5 kg.

Table 6-2

Length (cm)	Weight below which child is malnourished (kg)
60	4.6
61	4.9
62	5.2
63	5.4
64	5.6
65	6.0
66	6.2
67	6.4
68	6.7
69	6.9
70	7.2
71	7.5
72	7.8
73	8.0
74	8.2
75	8.4
76	8.6
77	8.8
78	9.0
79	9.2
80	9.4

• Activity 10 — Upper

• Looking at charts

Figures 6-16 and 6-17 show charts for two (imaginary) villages called Kijiji Cha Matiti and Kijiji Cha Chupa.

All the children in each village are marked on a health card. Each child is represented by a dot marked to show weight and age.

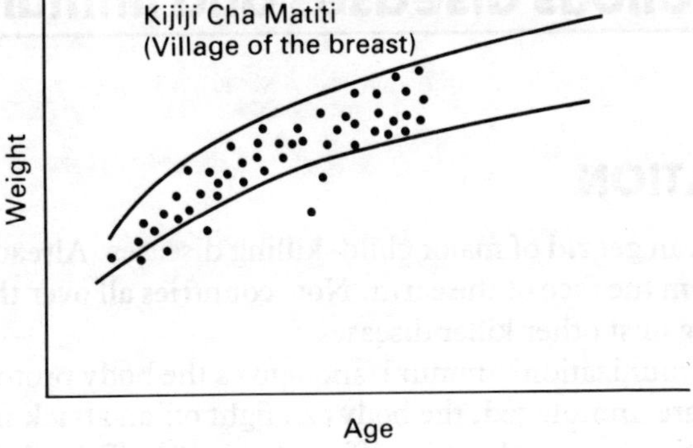

6-16 Weight–age chart for Kijiji Cha Matiti (village of the breast)

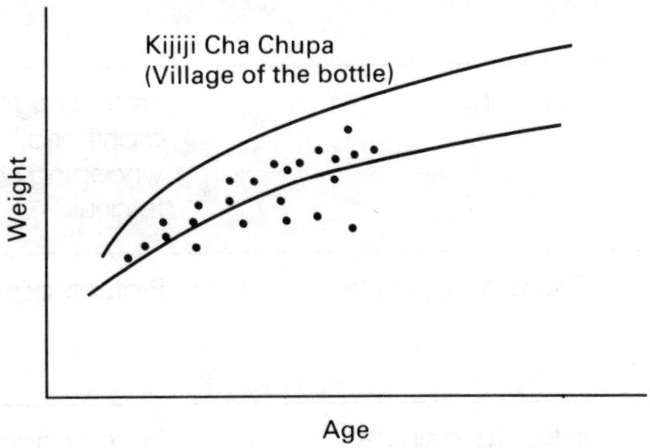

6-17 Weight–age chart for Kijiji Cha Chupa (village of the bottle)

Questions

Here are some questions that the children can answer on these two charts:

(1) How many children are malnourished in each village? (These children are shown by the dots below the bottom curve.)
(2) What is the percentage of malnourished children in each village?
(3) Which village has the higher number of children who are malnourished?
(4) Which village has the higher percentage of malnourished children?
(5) Which village has healthier children? Why?

7 Infectious diseases and immunization

IMMUNIZATION

Immunization can get rid of major child–killing diseases. Already smallpox has disappeared from the face of the earth. Now countries all over the world are fighting a war against other killer diseases.

What is immunization? Immunization gives the body protection against a disease. If you are immunized, the body can fight off an attack from the disease.

Immunization is carried out in different ways (see Table 7-1).

Table 7-1

DPT	Injections	Protects against diphtheria, whooping cough and tetanus
Polio vaccine	Drops in the mouth	Protects against polio
BCG	In Kenya, a single injection on the back of the left arm just below the elbow. In other countries it may be given in a different place.	Protects against tuberculosis (TB)
Measles	Single injection	Protects against measles

A child should have all these immunizations before the age of 9 months.

There are still some diseases which cannot be prevented by immunization, for example, ringworm, cancer, heart disease and AIDS.

But the success of immunization in saving lives and protecting children is enormous. The graph in figure 7-1 shows how immunization reduced the cases of polio in Brazil.

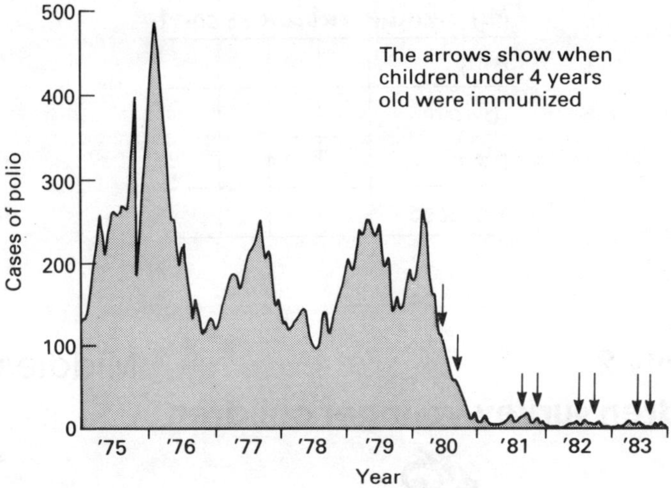

7-1 Graph showing decline of polio in Brazil due to immunization

Many immunization campaigns have been as successful as this one in Brazil. But still every 6 seconds (less time than it takes to read this sentence), one child dies and another is disabled from a disease which could be prevented by immunization.

The barriers to immunization are:

- the lack of effective vaccine,
- the attitude of parents.

Which of these barriers can you help to remove? Which can the children help to remove?

This chapter suggests mathematical activities which will increase the children's awareness of the diseases which can be prevented by immunization.

• Activity 1 — Middle

• Class survey

Carry out a survey of your class to find out which children have been immunized. To find out if they have had the BCG immunization, the children can look on their arms for the scar.

For the other immunizations the children will need to ask their parents. Let each child prepare a record to be filled in at home like the one in figure 7-2.

The children can then fill in a chart with their results.

My immunization record				
BCG				
Polio				
DPT				
Measles				

7-2

- Activity 2 — Middle/upper
- **Children survey younger children**

This should be an easier activity than Activity 1 as most parents of young children will have a health record card for the child (see figure 7-3). On this card there is a record of the immunizations the child has received.

CHILD'S NAME		GIRL / BOY
DATE OF BIRTH (day month year)	BIRTH WEIGHT	

MOTHER'S NAME	
CARETAKER IF NOT THE MOTHER	
FATHER'S NAME	
WHERE DOES THE CHILD LIVE?	

CARD GIVEN AND MOTHER TAUGHT BY	

IMMUNIZATIONS		DATE GIVEN
BCG		
POLIO	FIRST DOSE	
	SECOND DOSE	
	THIRD DOSE	
	FOURTH DOSE	
DPT (Diphtheria, Whooping Cough, Tetanus)	FIRST DOSE	
	SECOND DOSE	
	THIRD DOSE	
MEASLES		
MOTHER'S TETANUS TOXOID (or one booster)	FIRST DOSE	
	SECOND DOSE	
	THIRD DOSE	

ORAL REHYDRATION DATES			
Taught			
Used			

7-3 Child's health record card

Your class can carry out a survey of all children between the ages of 1 and 5 years in their households.

The children can ask the parents to tell them which immunizations each child has received, or they can read the information from the child's health record card.

Child's name	Age	BCG	Polio	DPT	Measles
Malindi	4	✓	✓	×	×
Ruth	3	✓	✓	✓	✓

7-4 Immunization record for my younger brother and sister

Figure 7-4 shows an example of the way children can record the information.

Then the results collected by each child can be filled in on a class chart like the one in figure 7-5.

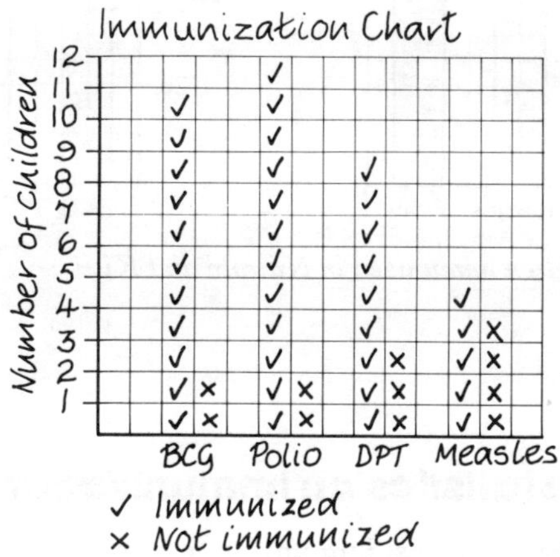

7-5

There will be many mathematical questions you can ask about the chart. For example,

- How many children in the survey were immunized against polio?
- What percentage of the children have been immunized against measles?
- What fraction of the children were immunized against polio?

• Activity 3 — Upper

• Comparing with national data

The Ministry of Health in many countries carries out surveys like that described in Activity 2. For Kenya, for example, here are the charts that show the percentage of children immunized in two areas (figure 7-6).

If the children calculate the percentage of children in their survey who are immunized, they can compare their percentages with those shown in these graphs (figure 7-6).

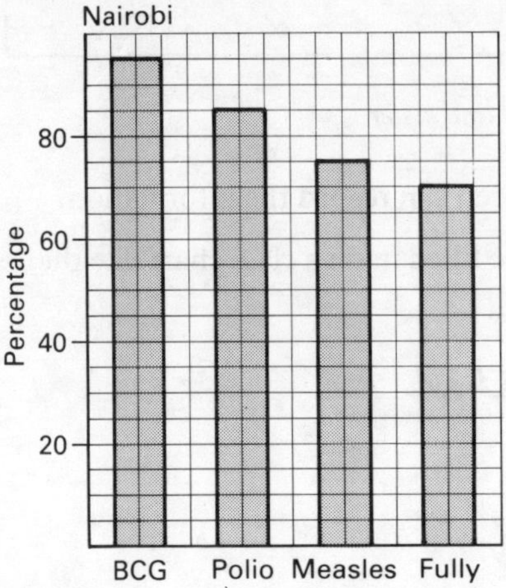

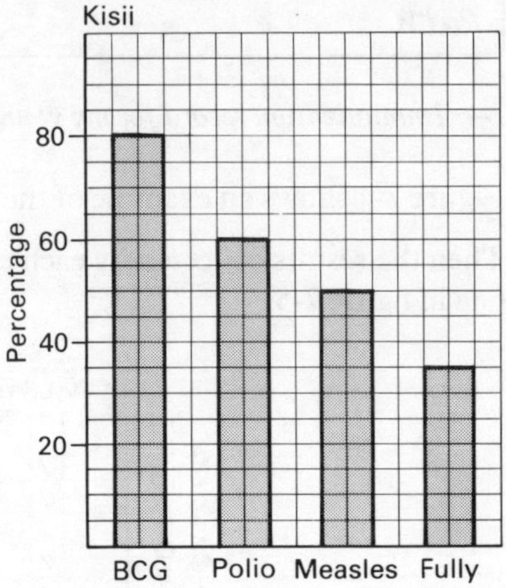

7-6 Percentage of children immunized in Nairobi and Kisii

• Activity 4 Upper

• Looking at statistics on immunization

Interpreting graphs based on past immunization campaigns helps children to learn how effective immunization can be. Here are some simplified data that children can show on a graph and then answer questions about.

Exercise 1 Table 7-2

Year	Cases of whooping cough in Fiji
1950	50
1952	250
1954	120
1956	180
1958	300
1960	120
1962	150
1964	500
1968	40
1970	10
1972	0

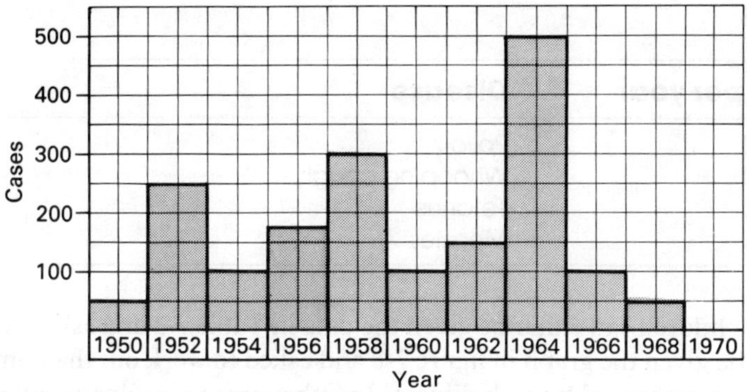

7-7 Chart showing cases of whooping cough in Fiji

Here are some sample questions on Table 7-2 and figure 7-7.

- How many cases of whooping cough were there in 1960?
- What year had the greatest number of cases?
- How many more cases of whooping cough were there in 1964 than 1962?
- When was whooping cough wiped out?
- How was whooping cough wiped out?

Exercise 2
The graph in figure 7-8 demonstrates the number of deaths that are still caused each year by diseases which can be prevented by immunization.

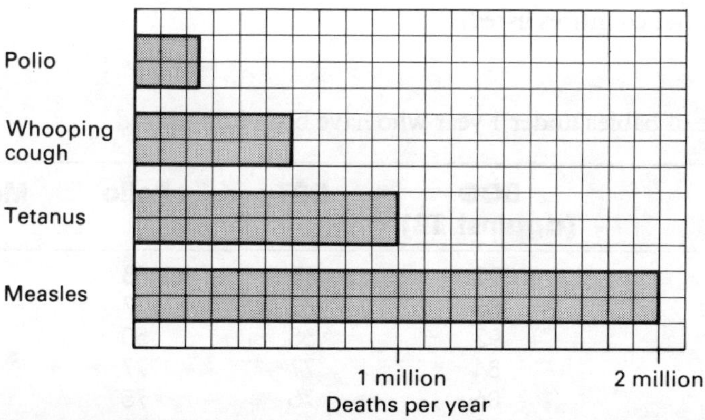

7-8 Deaths in the world per year from diseases which can be prevented by immunization

Table 7-3

Deaths per year	Disease
250 000	Polio
600 000	Whooping cough
1 000 000	Tetanus
2 000 000	Measles

The children can either be given the data in Table 7-3 and asked to plot a graph or be given the graph in figure 7-8 and asked to work out the number of deaths per year caused by each disease. In either case the children will need help in working out the scale.

• Activity 5 Upper

• Reading information from a table

Table 7-4 shows immunization information from many countries. The children can practise reading information from the table. Here are some sample questions.

- What percentage of babies under one are immunized against measles in Kenya?
- Which country has 50% of children under one immunized against polio?
- Which immunization has least coverage in Zimbabwe?
- Is this also true for Zambia?
- What kind of immunization has been most successful (a) in Botswana (b) in all the other countries listed?

Table 7-4
Percentage of babies under 1 year who have been immunized.

	BCG (against TB)	DPT	Polio	Measles
Botswana	99	86	88	91
Zimbabwe	86	77	77	73
Malawi	92	55	50	53
Lesotho	84	77	77	79
Kenya	86	75	75	60
Tanzania	95	81	80	78
Zambia	92	66	61	58
Uganda	74	39	40	48

The children can display the percentage shown in Table 7-4 as numbers in the form of percentage pictures. Each percentage can be shown by shading a 10 by 10 square. For example, the percentage immunized in Botswana can be shown like this (figure 7-9):

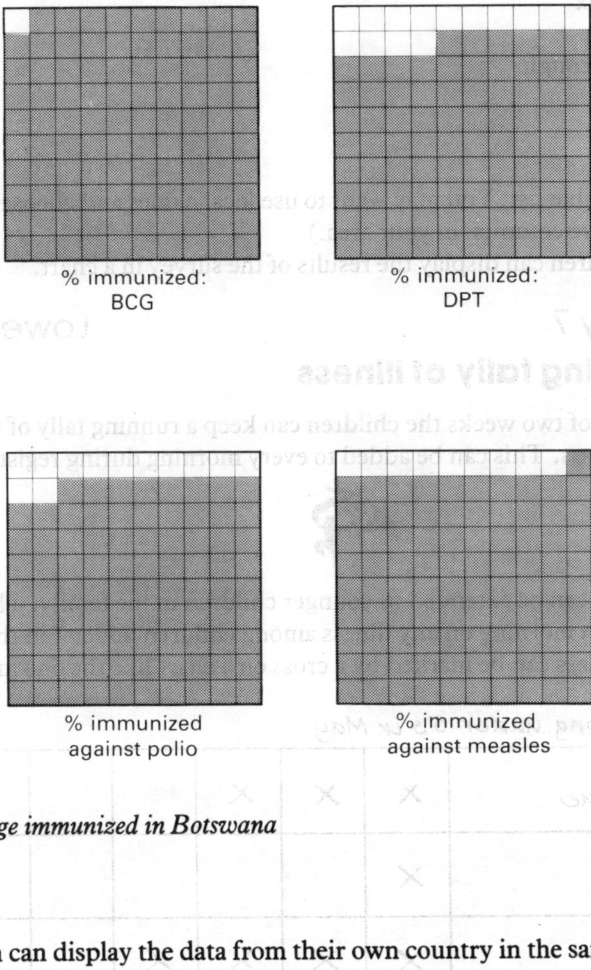

7-9 Percentage immunized in Botswana

The children can display the data from their own country in the same way.

INFECTIOUS DISEASES

Immunization has done much to prevent children dying from infectious diseases. Many children will have suffered from diseases which are spread by close contact, water or insects. The next section aims to make the children aware of these diseases and to give a mathematical illustration of the way they spread.

• Activity 6 Lower/middle

• Illness survey

Conduct a class survey of illnesses the child may have had. Find out if the children have had:

- Chicken pox
- Measles
- Whooping cough
- Malaria
- Ringworm
- Red eye

(This is a possible list. You may want to use local names and choose different diseases that are common in your area.)

The children can display the results of the survey in a chart.

• Activity 7 Lower/middle

• A running tally of illness

Over a period of two weeks the children can keep a running tally of the illness within their class. This can be added to every morning during registration.

This idea can be extended to younger children in the family. The children can report each morning on any illness among children under 5 in their home. Each day's illness can be marked by a cross on a chart like the one in figure 7-10.

Illness among under 5s in May

	1	2	3	4	5	6	7
Stomachache	×	×	×				
Fever	×						
Diarrhoea	×	×	×	×			
Measles							
Whooping cough	×						

Number of children

7-10

• Activity 8 Lower/middle

• Hand touching models the way disease spreads

This game is a simulation or model of the way infectious diseases spread.

How to play
All the children close their eyes and you touch one child. This child starts off with the 'disease'. The 'disease' is shown by holding the thumb tucked into the palm (see figure 7-11).

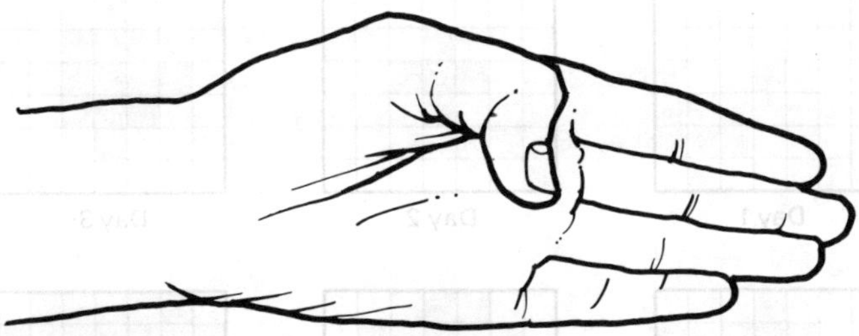

7-11 'Bent thumb' disease

Now each child touches hands with another child. The child who touches the 'bent thumb' now also has the disease and must also bend the thumb. Once again each child touches hands with another child. Any child who touches a 'bent thumb' catches the disease. Continue and see how quickly every child catches 'bent thumb' disease.

Repeat the game starting with a different child but this time find out after each round of hand touching how many have caught the disease. Fill in the results on the board.

The children can guess how many rounds it will take for the whole class to catch 'bent thumb' disease.

Encourage the children to guess how many rounds it will take for the disease to spread through larger groups. Let them test out their ideas when two or more classes are combined.

Variation

Now 'immunize' some of the children by giving them an imaginary injection against 'bent thumb' disease. These children will not catch the 'bent thumb' even though they touch a child with it. Play the game again and let the children record the number with the disease after each round. Investigate with the class the effect of increasing immunization.

• Activity 9 Lower/middle

• The touching squares show how disease spreads

This is another activity to illustrate the way disease spreads.

Each child draws a 7 × 7 square on squared paper and colours the middle square. This square has a disease. This is day 1.

The next day, day 2, any square touching the coloured one catches the disease. Now 5 squares will be coloured (see figure 7-12).

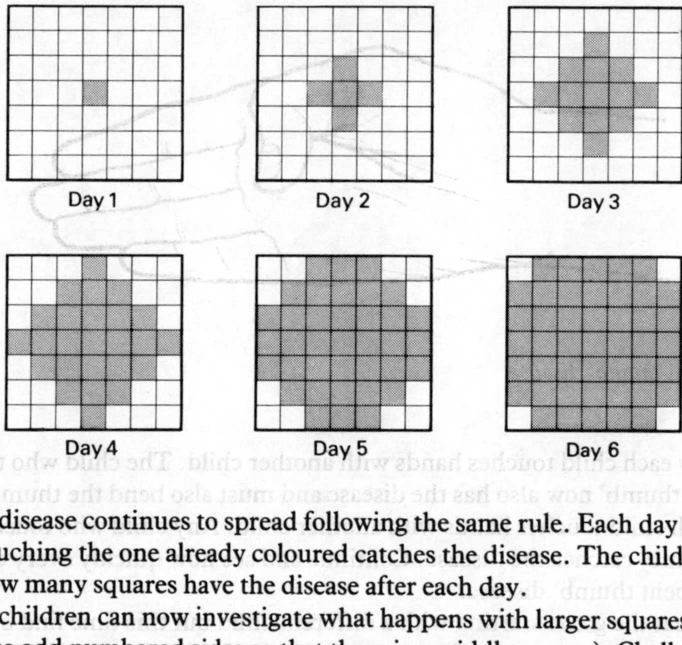

7-12

The disease continues to spread following the same rule. Each day any square touching the one already coloured catches the disease. The children record how many squares have the disease after each day.

The children can now investigate what happens with larger squares than 7 × 7, (use odd numbered sides so that there is a middle square). Challenge them to predict how many days a 9 × 9 square will take to fill. Then let them check their guess by colouring. What happens with an 11 × 11 square or a 5 × 5 square?

Discuss with the children how the spread of coloured squares is like the spread of common infectious diseases. Colds, ringworm and measles can spread rapidly through the school starting with just one person.

Immunization and touching squares

After the children have investigated what happens on larger diagrams you can suggest they see what happens if some of the squares are 'immunized'.

A cross inside a square in figure 7-13 means that it is immunized and will not be affected by touching squares. The children can try 'immunizing' squares of their own choice to see how this affects the spread of the 'disease'.

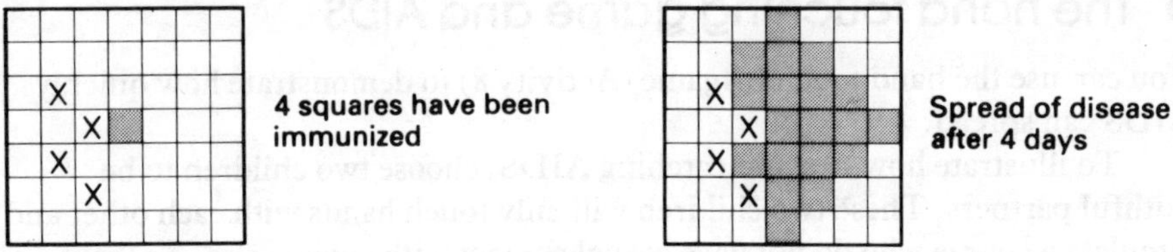

7-13

• Activity 10 Upper
• AIDS

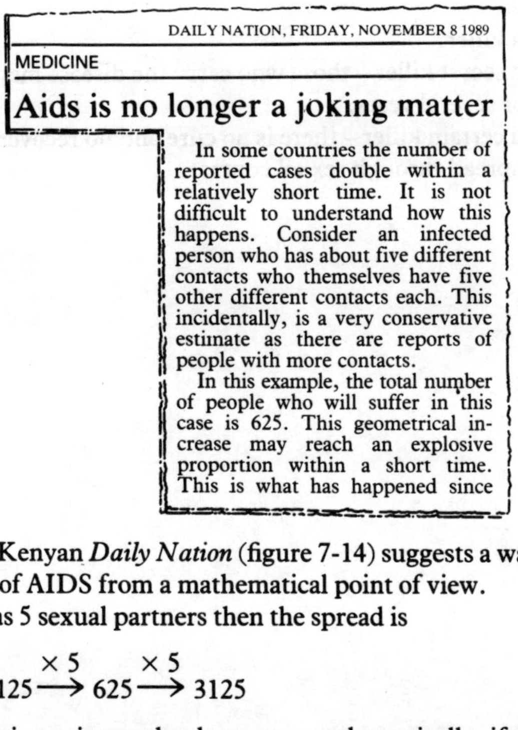

DAILY NATION, FRIDAY, NOVEMBER 8 1989

MEDICINE

Aids is no longer a joking matter

In some countries the number of reported cases double within a relatively short time. It is not difficult to understand how this happens. Consider an infected person who has about five different contacts who themselves have five other different contacts each. This incidentally, is a very conservative estimate as there are reports of people with more contacts.

In this example, the total number of people who will suffer in this case is 625. This geometrical increase may reach an explosive proportion within a short time. This is what has happened since

7-14

This report from the Kenyan *Daily Nation* (figure 7-14) suggests a way of looking at the spread of AIDS from a mathematical point of view.

If each person has 5 sexual partners then the spread is

$$1 \xrightarrow{\times 5} 5 \xrightarrow{\times 5} 25 \xrightarrow{\times 5} 125 \xrightarrow{\times 5} 625 \xrightarrow{\times 5} 3125$$

The children can investigate what happens, mathematically, if there are 4 partners, or 6 partners, or 2 partners.

$$1 \xrightarrow{\times 4} 4 \xrightarrow{\times 4} 16 \xrightarrow{\times 4} ? \xrightarrow{\times 4} ? \xrightarrow{\times 4} ? \xrightarrow{\times 4} ?$$

$$1 \xrightarrow{\times 6} 6 \longrightarrow 36 \longrightarrow ? \longrightarrow ? \longrightarrow ? \longrightarrow ?$$

$$1 \xrightarrow{\times 2} ? \longrightarrow ? \longrightarrow ? \longrightarrow ? \longrightarrow ? \longrightarrow ?$$

What happens if each person has one partner?

$$1 \xrightarrow{\times 1} ? \longrightarrow ? \longrightarrow ? \longrightarrow ? \longrightarrow ? \longrightarrow ?$$

• The hand touching game and AIDS

You can use the hand touching game (Activity 8) to demonstrate how quickly AIDS can spread.

To illustrate how to avoid catching AIDS, choose two children to be faithful partners. These two children will only touch hands with each other and simulate a couple who do not have sexual contact with anyone else. As 'bent thumb' disease spreads throughout the class these two children will stay healthy.

There are four things to remember about AIDS:

- AIDS is a killer.
- AIDS is a secret killer – those who carry the disease may have no marks of disease for several years.
- AIDS is a certain killer – there is no cure and no recovery.
- AIDS is spread through sexual contact.

8 Treating diarrhoea: the sugar–salt solution

Diarrhoea is the main cause of death in young children. The continued loss of water from the body due to repeated watery stools leads to dehydration. If a plant is dehydrated it loses strength and dies. It is the same with young children (see figure 8-1).

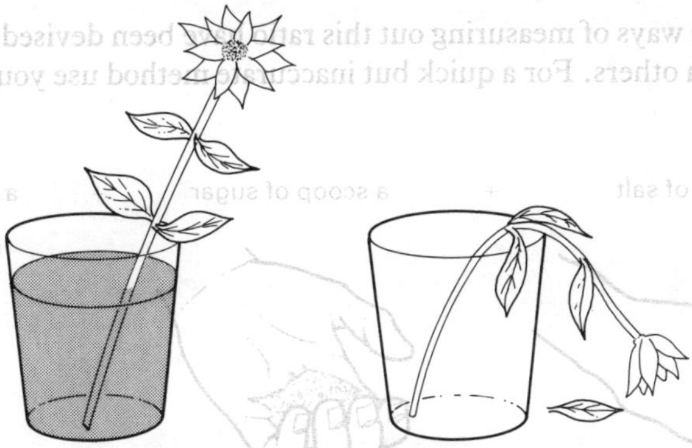

Dehydration kills plants

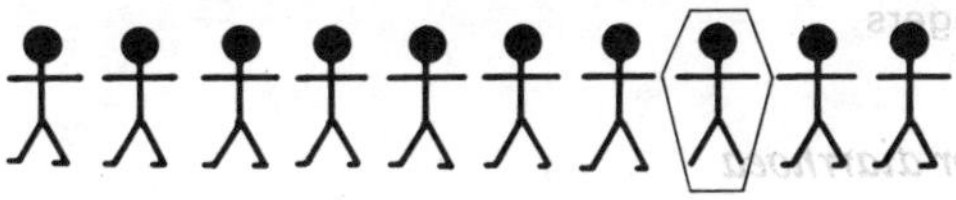

8-1 It also kills one child in ten

It is estimated that in the first five years of life *each* child has 10 attacks of diarrhoea.

One child in ten is likely to die from the dehydration caused by diarrhoea. But there is a safe, simple and cheap cure for dehydration, simple enough for a primary school child to learn and use. It involves simple ideas of measurement and ratio.

It is called the sugar–salt solution. Teaching children how to make the sugar–salt solution will help them learn practical mathematics and could save lives. If they learn about the sugar-salt solution at school, they can go home and make the sugar–salt solution for a younger child with diarrhoea.

What is the sugar–salt solution?
Diarrhoea leads to the loss of much fluid from the body. The sugar–salt solution is a drink that helps to put fluid back into the body.

How does the sugar–salt solution work?
During diarrhoea the body loses salt and water. Drinking a mixture of salt, sugar and water will help replace the salt and water the body has lost. The sugar helps to carry salt into the body.

How is the sugar–salt solution made?
For the solution to work well as a medicine, the sugar, salt and water must be mixed in the correct ratio.

The correct ratio is:

1 part of salt : 8 parts of sugar : 200 parts of water.

Many simple ways of measuring out this ratio have been devised. Some are more accurate than others. For a quick but inaccurate method use your hands (see figure 8-2).

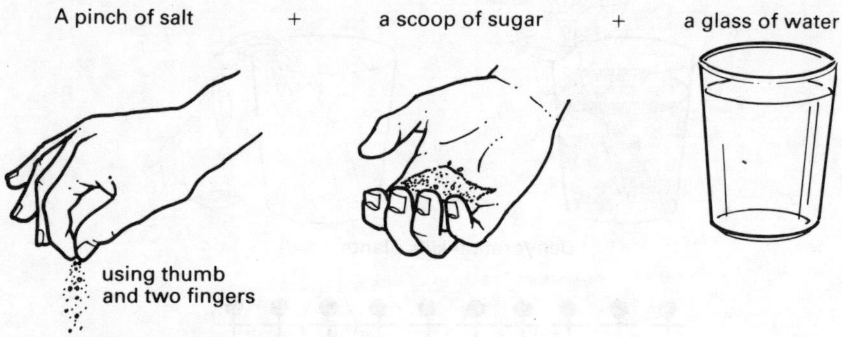

8-2 Making a cure for diarrhoea

or a teaspoon:

tip of teaspoon of salt + a teaspoon of sugar + a glass of water

or bottle-tops:

½ bottle-top of salt + 4 bottle-tops of sugar + 1 litre of water

A more accurate way to measure the salt and sugar is to use cups made by folding paper. This is a good method to teach in the primary school and is fully described in Activity 5 on page 128.

Using paper cups to make the sugar–salt solution, the proportions are:

small paper cup of salt + larger paper cup of sugar + a glass of water

How much sugar–salt solution should be given?
A child with diarrhoea needs 1 glass of sugar–salt solution for every watery stool.

An adult with diarrhoea needs 2 glasses of sugar–salt solution for every watery stool.

• Activity 1 Middle/upper

• A survey of the occurrence of diarrhoea

A survey of how often children suffer from diarrhoea will help them to see how common a problem it is. Make a chart of the number of children who have had diarrhoea

in the last week
in the last month
in the last term
in the last year
in their lives sometime

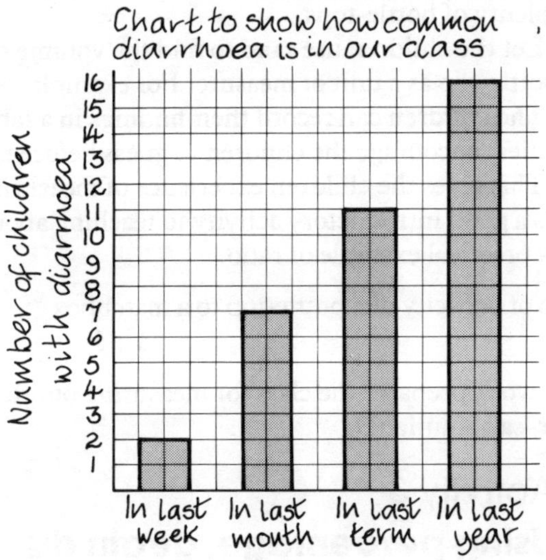

8-3

An alternative activity is to keep a tally chart throughout the term like the one in figure 8-4. The children can fill in on the chart any cases of diarrhoea in their homes, especially among younger brothers and sisters.

If you keep this chart going while you teach about the sugar–salt solution, then the children can also record the number of times they have helped make a sugar–salt solution in their homes to cure dehydration.

Tally chart showing children in our homes with diarrhoea

	Number of children with diarrhoea
Week 1	✓ ✓ ✓ ✓
Week 2	✓ ✓ ✓ ✓ ✓ ✓ ✓
Week 3	✓ ✓ ✓ ✓ ✓
Week 4	✓ ✓ ✓ ✓ ✓ ✓ ✓ ✓
Week 5	
Week 6	

8-4

• Activity 2 Middle

• Capacity and volume, measuring with bottle-tops

Collect a variety of different sized containers, lids, match boxes, cups, small tins and plenty of bottle-tops.

Let the children use sand to find the volume of each of the containers using the bottle-top as a unit of measure. For example, 5-bottle-tops fill a match box.

The children can record their findings in a table. As with all measurement activities, encourage the children to guess before measuring.

This gives the children experience of measuring the capacity of containers and is a good introductory activity to teaching about litres and millilitres. It is also a practical example of ratio.

Ratio of capacity of a bottle-top to a matchbox

1 : 5

Such work prepares the class for measuring out the salt and sugar for the sugar–salt solution.

• Activity 3 Upper

• Using percentage, death due to diarrhoea

This activity aims to make children aware that diarrhoea is a common cause of death and to give practice in using percentages.

Each child draws around a 10 by 10 square on squared paper. The children draw a picture of a child in each square.

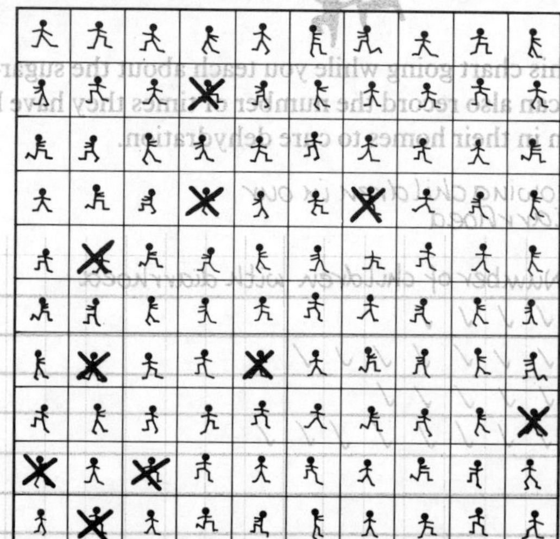

8-5 Chart to show percentage of children who have died due to diarrhoea

Then ask them to cross out any 10 of the children (figure 8-5). This represents the death of a child due to diarrhoea. Ask them what percentage of children have died.

An exercise using percentage

From the exercise above the children have learnt that 10% of children die due to diarrhoea. Table 8-1 shows the number of children living in various towns and districts of Kenya. Ask the children to calculate the number of children who are likely to die from diarrhoea.

Table 8-1

Place	Number of children born	Number of children likely to die from diarrhoea
Samburu	1 900	$\frac{10}{100} \times 1900 = 190$
Nyeri	24 320	
Lamu	1 540	
Isiolo	1 820	

• Activity 4 — Upper

• Ratios, the sugar-salt solution

Ask each child to bring a litre bottle so they can each make up a sugar–salt solution.

First demonstrate how to measure out the salt and the sugar using bottle-tops (see page 124) and then how to mix it with the litre of water. If possible the water should be boiled to make it clean and safe. Let the children make up their own solutions. Let them taste them. Let each child record how the solution was made and how it is to be used.

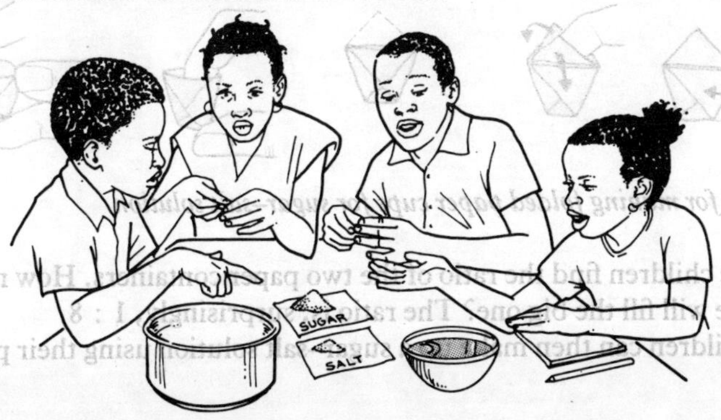

8-6 Making the sugar–salt solution

Further exercise on making the sugar–salt solution
Put the class in groups and give each group a container which is not 1 litre but is larger or smaller. Set the children the problem of deciding how much salt and sugar they should add to this new container so that the sugar–salt solution is still made in the correct ratio (figure 8-6).

Example: A container holding 500 ml should have ¼ bottle-top of salt and 2 bottle-tops of sugar.

• Activity 5 Upper

• Ratios, paper cups for sugar-salt solution

Here is a very practical and mathematical way for children to make measuring cups for salt and sugar. The cups will be the right size for making one glass of sugar–salt solution.

Each child will need a square of paper of size 6 cm. They can draw this on squared paper and then cut it out.

Then get them to fold it following the method in figure 8-7. Practise how to do this first yourself, then demonstrate to the children using a very large square of paper (e.g. from a square of newspaper).

To make the cup for the salt, the children will need to cut squares of size 3 cm. This is folded in exactly the same way.

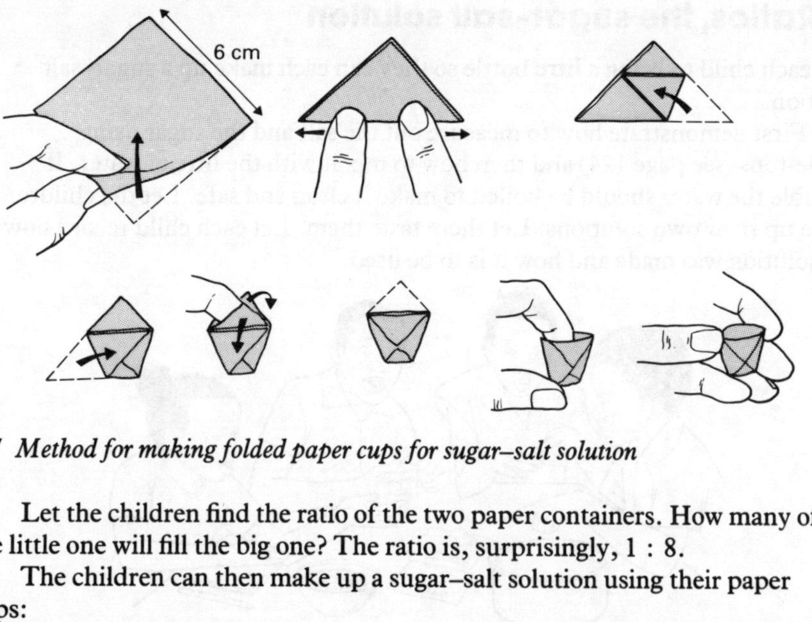

8-7 Method for making folded paper cups for sugar–salt solution

Let the children find the ratio of the two paper containers. How many of the little one will fill the big one? The ratio is, surprisingly, 1 : 8.

The children can then make up a sugar–salt solution using their paper cups:

Small paper cup of salt + larger paper cup of sugar + a glass of water

• Activity 6 Upper

• Statistics on ORT

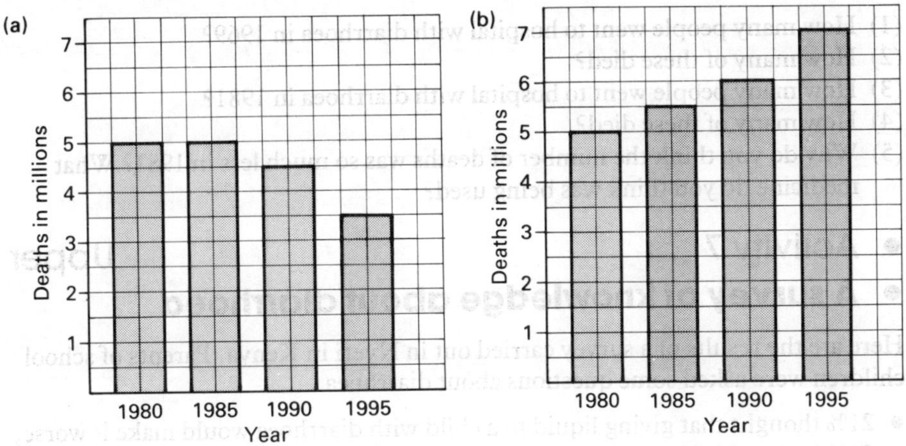

8-8 (a) Child deaths if ORT is used (b) Child deaths if ORT is not used

Health clinics and hospitals use a special solution to cure dehydration. It acts like the sugar–salt solution and is called Oral Rehydration Therapy or ORT.

Exercise 1

Sample questions on figure 8-8:

(1) How many children will die in 1990 if ORT is not used?
(2) How many children will die in 1990 if ORT is used?
(3) How many lives can be saved in 1990 by using ORT?

Exercise 2

The graph in figure 8-9 shows how many people with diarrhoea were admitted to Cuban hospitals.

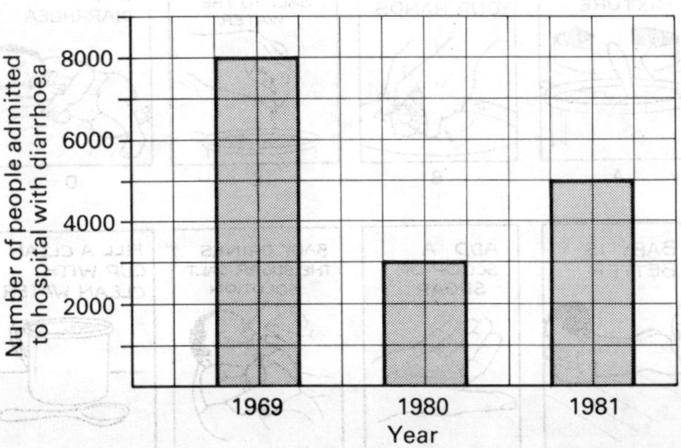

8-9 Graph showing number of people admitted to Cuban hospitals with diarrhoea

In 1969, 35% of those with diarrhoea died.
In 1981, 2% of those with diarrhoea died.
From the graph, answer the following questions.

(1) How many people went to hospital with diarrhoea in 1969?
(2) How many of these died?
(3) How many people went to hospital with diarrhoea in 1981?
(4) How many of these died?
(5) Why do you think the number of deaths was so much less in 1981? What medicine do you think was being used?

• Activity 7 **Upper**
• A survey of knowledge about diarrhoea

Here are the results of a survey carried out in Nyeri in Kenya. Parents of school children were asked some questions about diarrhoea.

- 21% thought that giving liquid to a child with diarrhoea would make it worse,
- 26% had no idea how diarrhoea was caused,
- 52% believed diarrhoea could not be passed from one person to another.

Find out what the children in your class believe about diarrhoea by carrying out a class survey. Discuss the results and suggest that the children survey their parents. Work out the percentages from the results.

• Activity 8 **Upper**
• A cure for diarrhoea, an exercise in ordering

Draw up the activities in figure 8–10 on the board and label the drawings.

Ask the children to arrange the boxes in the correct order.

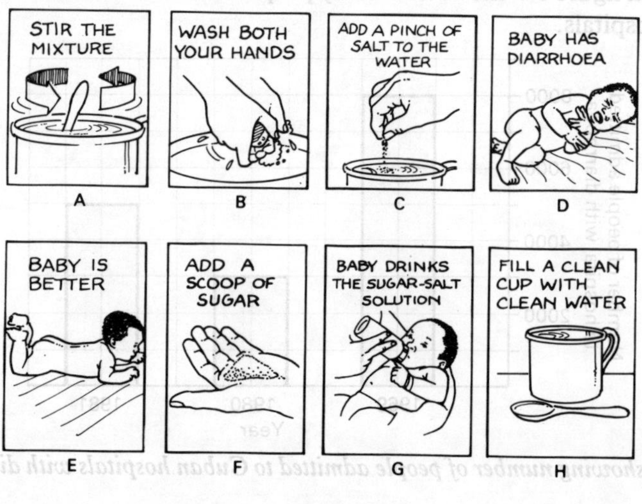
STIR THE MIXTURE
A
WASH BOTH YOUR HANDS
B
ADD A PINCH OF SALT TO THE WATER
C
BABY HAS DIARRHOEA
D
BABY IS BETTER
E
ADD A SCOOP OF SUGAR
F
BABY DRINKS THE SUGAR-SALT SOLUTION
G
FILL A CLEAN CUP WITH CLEAN WATER
H

8-10

9 Water and sanitation

Water is essential to life and to good health. Everyone needs water to drink and to keep clean. But many people, especially those in rural areas, do not have clean water.

In towns and cities, 80% have safe, clean water. In the rural areas, only 30% have safe, clean water.

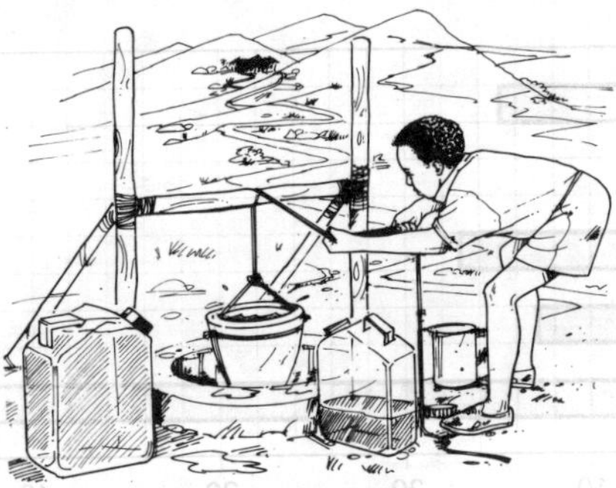

9-1 The well is a long way from this boy's village

Many people use very little water because they have to carry it a long way (figure 9-1). This often means that children are not kept clean and healthy.

Water is important in keeping the body healthy but it is also responsible for spreading disease. In Kenya, for example, there are over 25 diseases related to water. These diseases are:

- those spread through germs in the water, like diarrhoea,
- those spread through shortage of water, like skin disease,
- those spread through insects needing water to breed, like malaria and bilharzia.

These are some of the ways of preventing water being contaminated and spreading disease:

- Use a latrine. Do not urinate into a water source.
- Make sure latrines are built far from a water supply.
- Keep rubbish away from the water source.
- Clean the containers used to carry water.
- Cover the container in which water is kept in the house.
- Use a ladle or dipper to get out water for drinking.

The activities that follow should help to increase the children's awareness of the water they use. Do not miss any opportunity to slip in the health messages listed above.

• Activity 1 Middle/upper

• Comparing charts of water sources

If your school is in a rural area, then the children in your class will probably fetch water from many different sources: inside tap, outside tap, rain water, tank, spring, river, etc. The children can make a chart to show from where they fetch water.

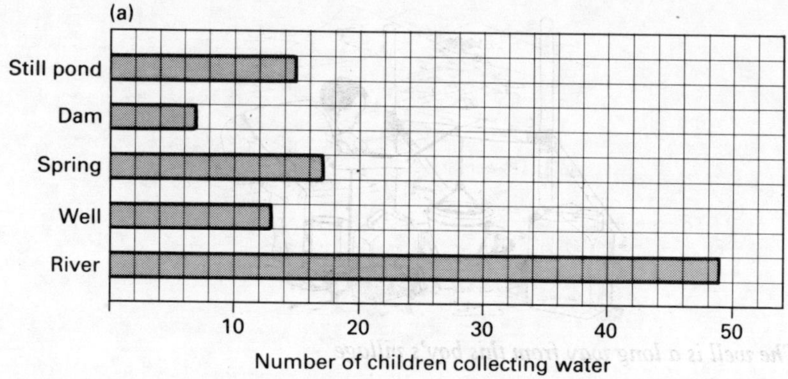

Figure 9-2(a) is an example of a chart which shows the different water sources used by children in the Baringo area of Kenya. The children can compare their chart with that of the Baringo children.

In Baringo, the sources of water vary at different times of the year. The chart in figure 9-2(a) shows the sources of water used in the wet season. The chart for the dry season is shown in figure 9-2(b).

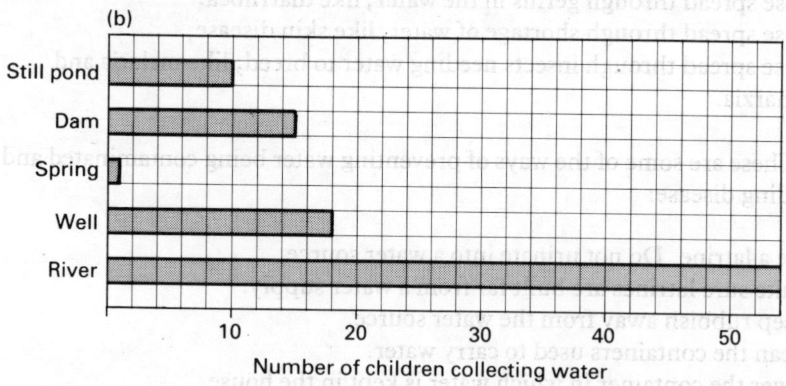

9-2 (a) Water sources used in Baringo (wet season) (b) Water sources used in Baringo (dry season)

Your class can make a dry season chart and a wet season chart for your area and compare them.

• Activity 2 Middle

• Capacity and weight of water containers

Children have first-hand experience of filling containers and carrying water to their homes. This provides a good basis for teaching about capacity and weight. Ideas about capacity come with the action of filling the containers from the well or tap.

Here are some suggestions about how to make use of this everyday experience.

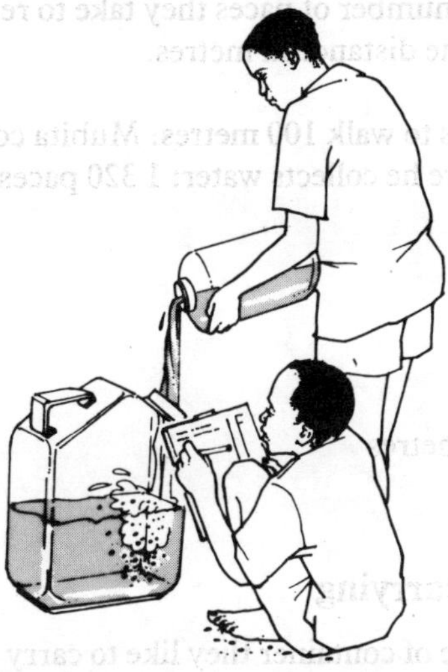

9-3 Measuring the volume of a container using a one-litre bottle

- Every child can bring from home a container used to carry water.
- Let the children measure some of the containers. They can use a one-litre bottle to fill them with water (figure 9-3).
- Encourage the children to guess the capacity of the rest of the containers. Then they can measure and compare their guesses with the actual capacities.
- Each child can keep a record of the activity (figure 9-4).

Container	Capacity		Weight of water
	Guess	Measure	
Jezra's can	5 litres	6 litres	6 kg

9-4

The weight column in figure 9-4 can be filled in by the children using the simple rule:

1 litre of water weighs 1 kg

• Activity 3 Upper

• Measuring distance from a water supply

The journey to collect water is often one of the most regular distances that children walk. When introducing the concept of measuring distance in kilometres, ask the children to estimate the distance they go to fetch water.

The children can find out how many of their normal paces make up 100 metres.

The children can count the number of paces they take to reach the source of water. Then they can calculate the distance in metres.

Example: Mubita takes 120 paces to walk 100 metres. Mubita counts the number of paces to the well where he collects water: 1 320 paces.

120 paces are 100 metres

1 pace is $\frac{100}{120}$ metres

1 320 paces are $\left(\frac{100}{120} \times 1320\right)$ metres

or 1 100 metres

Further activity on water carrying

Discuss with the children the size of container they like to carry when fetching water. Is it better to use a small container and make many journeys or a large container and fewer journeys?

Here is a situation for children to investigate.

Paulus has a choice of containers which can hold 1,2,4, or 6 litres. Each day he has to fetch 20 litres of water. Find all the ways he could fetch the water.

• Activity 4 Middle

• Statistics on how we use water

The children can list all the uses of water in their household and estimate how many litres they use for activities such as

- drinking
- cooking
- washing dishes
- bathing
- washing clothes

Table 9-1 gives some statistics of water use in two different Mozambiquan villages.

Table 9-1

	Average water use per day per person Village A	Village B
Drinking	200 ml	400 ml
Cooking	600 ml	1800 ml
Washing dishes	400 ml	1400 ml
Bathing	700 ml	4900 ml
Bathing children	100 ml	1200 ml
Washing clothes	500 ml	300 ml

Sample questions

(1) What was the total amount of water used per person in (a) Village A (b) Village B?
(2) What is the ratio of total water use per person in Village A to Village B?
(3) What is the ratio of drinking water volume in Village A to Village B?
(4) What are the ratios for all the other activities?
(5) In which activity is there the greatest difference in water use?
(6) Which village do you think is closest to its water source?
(7) Which village do you think is healthier?

Some extra information about the two villages

Villagers in Village A take 5 hours to fetch water. In Village B the time is only 15 minutes. Notice how little water is used in Village A for bathing children. The number of cases of trachoma (red eye leading to blindness) in Village A was twice that in Village B. This was because the children in Village B were washed well and often and those in Village A were not.

• Activity 5 — Middle/upper

• From source to mouth, a flow chart

Many diseases are spread through water and because the containers used to carry water are not clean. A valuable exercise in ordered and logical thinking is for children to trace the route of the water they drink from source to mouth. They can discover how many different containers the water passes through and how many chances of infection there are.

An example of a flow chart for the route of drinking water from well to mouth is shown in figure 9-5.

Discuss with the class the differences between their flow charts.

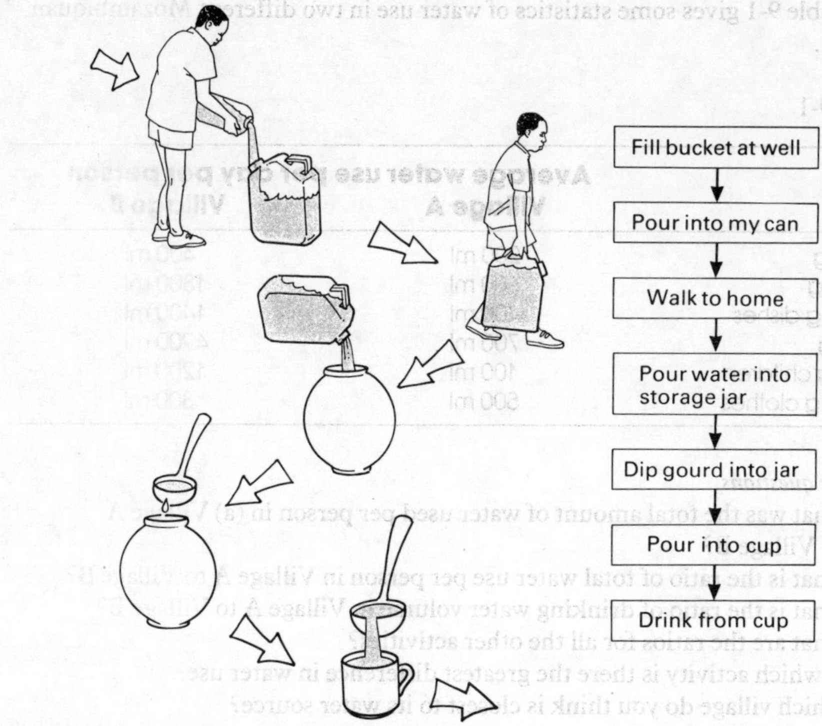

9-5 Flow chart of water collection and use

Further suggestions

- **Class survey to find how many boil their water before drinking. The children can find the ratio of those who do to those who do not.**
- **Class survey to find how the water is stored in the house; jar, can, bowl.**
- **Class survey to find how many keep the water container covered to keep off flies.**

• Activity 6 — Middle

• Toilet survey

First carry out a survey of the class to find which kind of toilets they use. Here is a possible list:

- **VIP (ventilated improved latrine)**
- **pit latrine**
- **water closet**
- **the bush**

Children in some schools have carried out a survey of the forms of sanitation used by different households in their village. An example of such a survey made up into a chart is shown in figure 9-6.

The children in your class can carry out a similar survey, make a chart of their results and compare it with the chart in figure 9-6.

You can use the results of the class survey as the starting point for a discussion with the class about ways of improving sanitation.

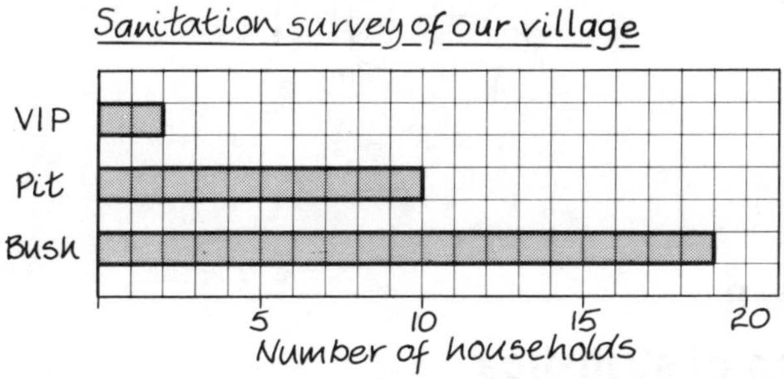

9-6

• Activity 7 Upper

• Building a school latrine, measuring

The school should be a model of good health in practice.

As a school project it may be necessary to build a pit latrine. There is plenty of mathematics in such an activity.

Where should it be placed? To be safe it should be 20 metres from all houses, wells and springs (figure 9–7).

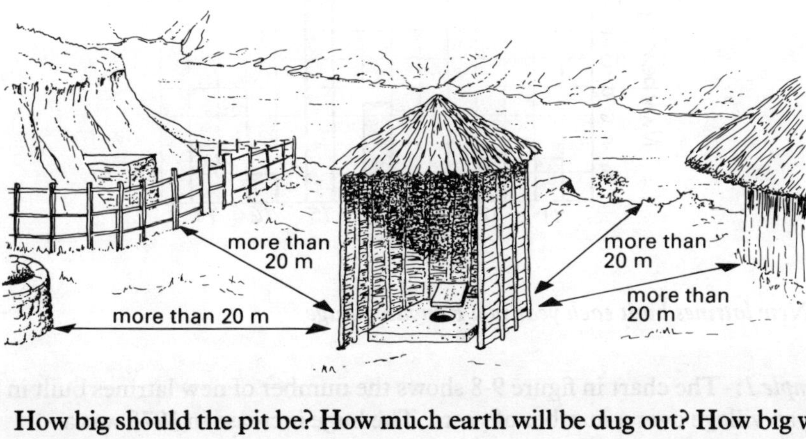

How big should the pit be? How much earth will be dug out? How big will the slab be?

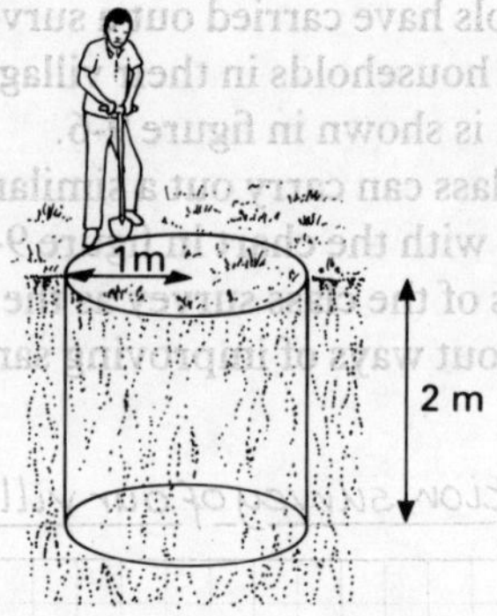

9-7

- **Activity 8** **Upper**
- **Looking at statistics**

Here are some statistics with a health message connected with them.

9-8 New latrines built each year in a Kenyan village

Example 1: The chart in figure 9-8 shows the number of new latrines built in a Kenyan village over a number of years. The huge increase in 1975 was a response to a cholera outbreak.

Example 2:

Table 9-2 Type of sewage disposal by provinces of Kenya

	Coast	Rift Valley	Western
Main sewer	2%	1%	0%
Septic tank	1%	1%	1%
Pit latrine	22%	32%	66%
Bucket latrine	0%	1%	0%
No sanitation	75%	65%	33%

Challenge the children to interpret the statistics in Table 9-2 and draw conclusions from them.

• Activity 9 Upper
• Using water meters to calculate water use

The activities so far listed have been suitable for rural schools. If most of your class have piped water and pay for it, you can ask them to bring to school old water bills. From the bills you can find the number of litres used. For example, a consumption of 24 000 litres means that 24 000 litres were used during the month. The children can then calculate the daily use per person.

Example: 24 000 litres used in 30 days.

Number of people in house = 10

$$\text{Average daily use} = \frac{24\,000}{30}\text{ litres}$$

$$\text{Average daily use per person} = \frac{24\,000}{30 \times 10} = 80\text{ litres}$$

The children can compare their daily use per person with others and explain where all the water goes.

• Activity 10 Upper
• Costing a water supply

As a class project the children can design and calculate the cost of a water supply for their village. Here are a few facts:

Cost of pipe per metre	=	5 shillings
Cost of pump	=	60 000 shillings
Cost of 40 000 litre tank	=	40 000 shillings
Cost of 60 000 litre tank	=	60 000 shillings

Example: A village is 6 km away from the dam. To build a water supply, one tank holding 40 000 litres, one pump and pipes will be needed. Cost of pipe from dam to village:

1 m of pipe costs 5 shillings
1000 m of pipe costs 5000 shillings
1 km of pipe costs 5000 shillings
6 km of pipe costs 30 000 shillings

total cost:

pipe	30 000 shillings
tank	40 000 shillings
pump	60 000 shillings
	130 000 shillings

The children can work out what a water supply would cost for their village by:

- working out how far it is to the water source
- working out if a pump and tank are necessary
- calculating the cost

10 The health of the growing mind

The priorities listed at the start of this book concentrate on ways of improving children's physical health. It must not be forgotten that the young child is growing in mind as well as in body.

A young child can be stunted in physical growth through poor nutrition. If bodily needs are not met then the child will not reach full height. In the same way, children whose mental needs are not satisfied will never reach their potential as human beings as their intellectual growth will be stunted.

In a research study done in South America, three groups of malnourished children from poor homes were given different kinds of care:

- *group 1* received medical care
- *group 2* received medical care and proper food
- *group 3* received medical care, proper food and a stimulating environment

The development of the children in each group was measured and compared with that of a group of elite children who already received medical care, proper food and a stimulating environment.

After two years, the first group was found to have no change in growth or intellect. The second group grew as well as the elite group but showed little change in intellect. The third group, however, showed the same growth in body and intellect as the elite group (see Table 10-1).

Table 10-1

		Change in growth	Change in intellect
Group 1	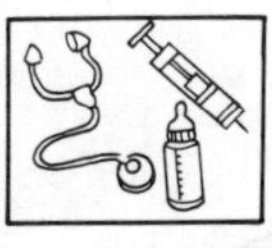	No	No
Group 2	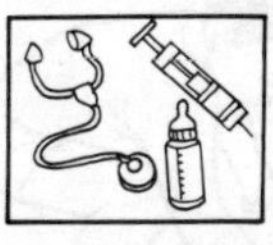 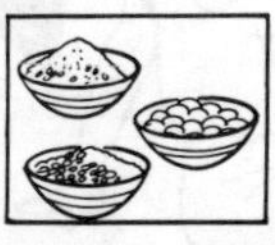	Yes	No
Group 3	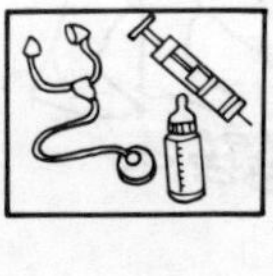 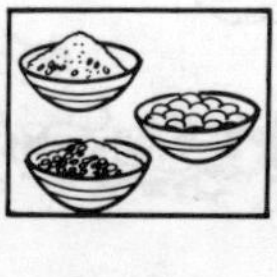 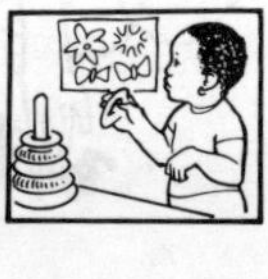	Yes	Yes

This evidence supports the belief that medical care and good nutrition are not enough to ensure full development of the young child. Lively and varied surroundings are also essential.

The first five years are vital, not just for the physical development of the child but for the mental development as well. Think of the amazing strides the child makes in the acquisition of language in those early years. It is easy to judge these achievements because we hear the child speak, we hear the single words become a phrase, the phrases become a sentence. At twelve months a child can give you an object you ask for. By four years of age a child can talk to you and can tell you what happened yesterday.

As well as learning language in the early years the child is also learning concepts and skills that will contribute to later mathematical understanding. Sorting by touch, feel, taste and appearance, comparing forms and colours, exploring their three-dimensional physical surroundings, all these activities help to create in the child's mind the conceptual foundations on which deeper understanding of shape and number can be built.

A child's learning of language depends on the richness of the verbal environment and a child deprived of sound will be stunted in language growth.

So too a child deprived of a stimulating physical environment will be slower to develop those foundations on which the early concepts of mathematics are based.

ENRICHING THE EARLY YEARS

Good health care means more than preventing illness and malnutrition in the young child. It also involves providing varied and stimulating learning experiences for the child.

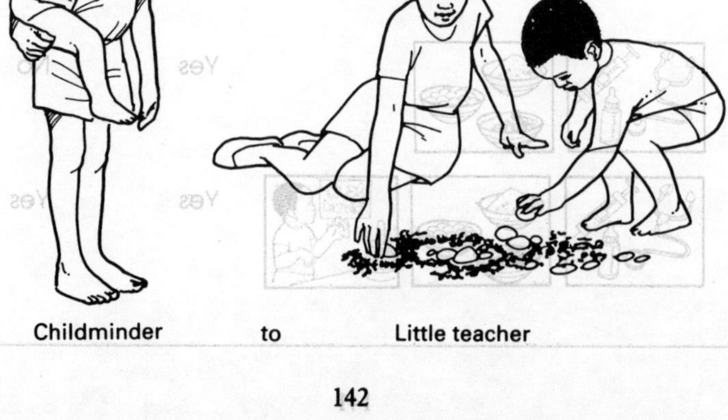

10-1

This is an aspect of health care in which primary school children can play a positive part. They spend much time caring for the young child at home, acting as a baby minder or comforter. Often this caring is of a passive kind, keeping the child contented and comfortable. But if these young child-minders can be encouraged to become little teachers, then they can do much to provide more enlivening experiences for the children in their care (see figure 10-1).

The activities that follow suggest some ways in which this change can be encouraged.

CLASSROOM ACTIVITIES AND CHILD-TO-CHILD ACTIVITIES

The activities suggested in this section are designed to fit into a teacher's normal lessons, to provide valuable learning experiences for the children in the class, but also to act as a stimulus for child-to-child activities, activities which the children can use with younger brothers and sisters when they go home from school.

• Activity 1 — Lower

• Teach maths facts with cat and rat

Class activity

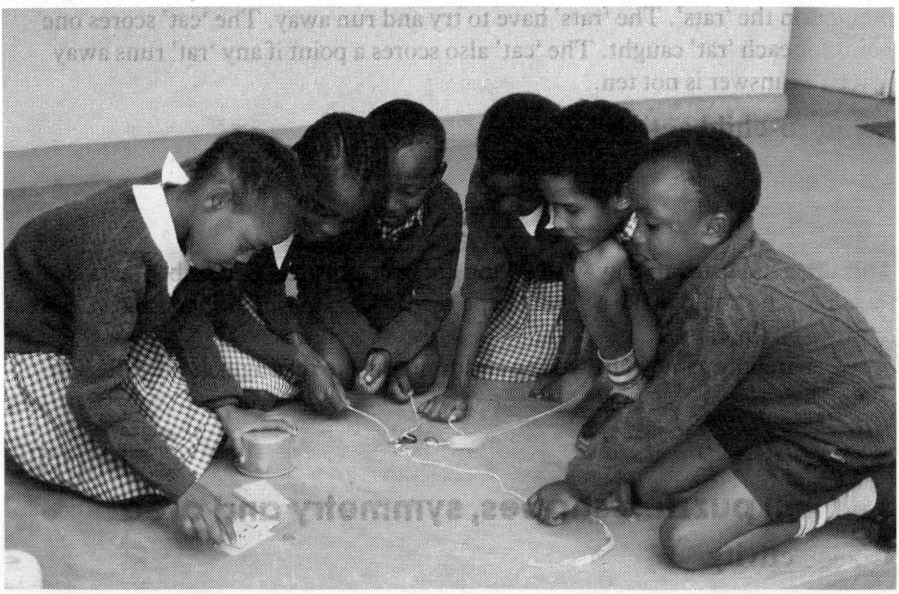

Plate 3 A game of 'Cat and rat'

This game can be used for learning a variety of number facts.

Children play in groups of about six. Each child needs a bottle-top with a 'tail' of string tied to it about 30 cm long. This is a 'rat'. Each group needs a 'cat'. A tin or plastic cup will do for this.

If the game is aimed at learning addition facts then the children should make a set of addition cards like the ones in figure 10-2.

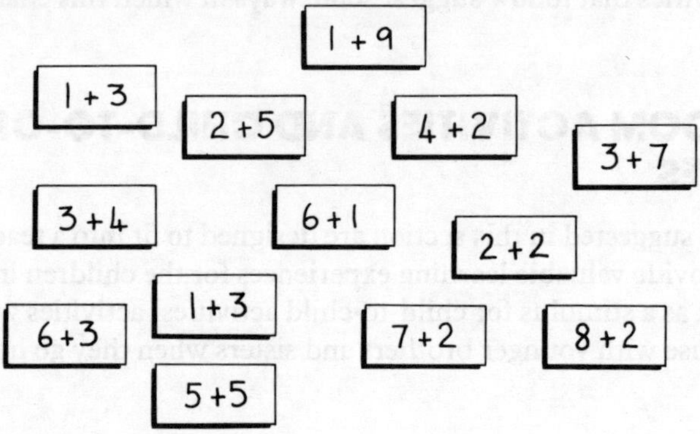

10-2 Addition cards for 'Cat and rat'

To play the game, put the cards in a pile. One child holds the 'cat' and all the others put their 'rats' close together holding on to the tail (see plate 3). The cards are turned over one at a time. If a card comes with *a sum of ten* the 'cat' can pounce on the 'rats'. The 'rats' have to try and run away. The 'cat' scores one point for each 'rat' caught. The 'cat' also scores a point if any 'rat' runs away when the answer is not ten.

Child-to-child activity

This is a good game to play with young children. Instead of number facts cards the children should make a set of shape cards. Decide which shape allows the cat to jump on the rats.

Playing the game helps young children learn to distinguish the different shapes.

• Activity 2 Middle

• Kumi puzzles, shapes, symmetry and area

Class activity

Here is an educational puzzle that can be made from an old matchbox. It helps children learn about shapes, symmetry and area.

Each child will need the outside of an old matchbox. Flatten the box. It makes a square. Draw a line from corner to corner.

Cut along this line to make two pieces. Open them out to give two triangles.

(a)

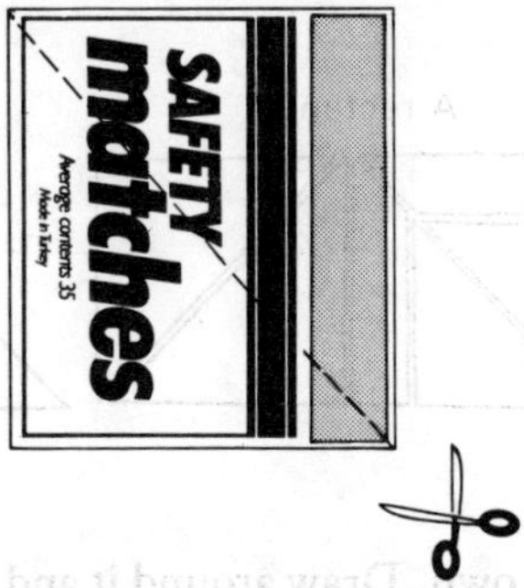

On each triangle you will see two long creases. Cut along these to give three pieces from each triangle.

(b)

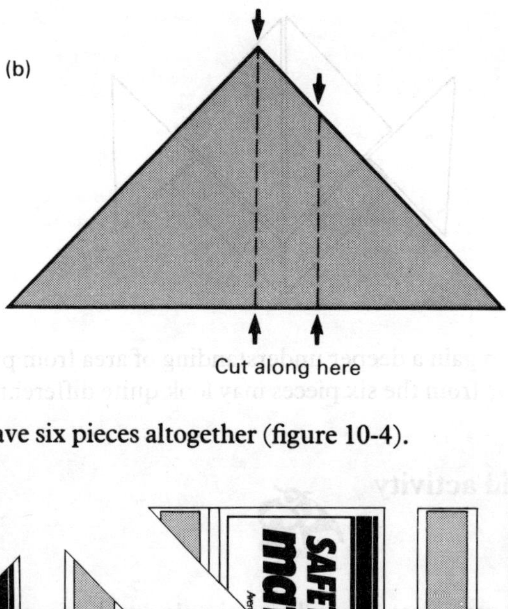

10-3

You should have six pieces altogether (figure 10-4).

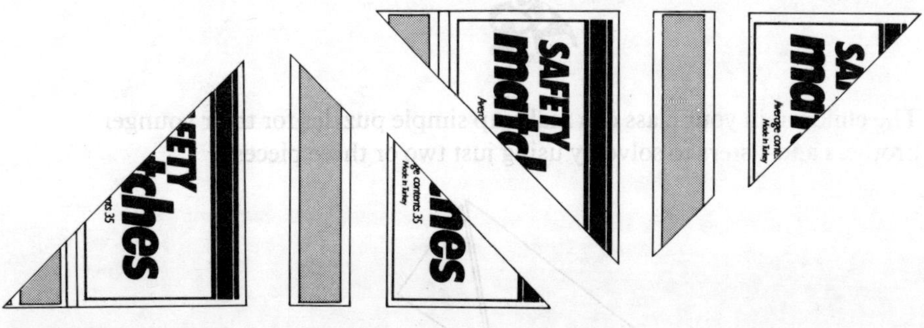

10-4

Puzzles for school children

Can you arrange the six pieces to make a square, a rectangle and a triangle? The answers can be found in figure 10-5.

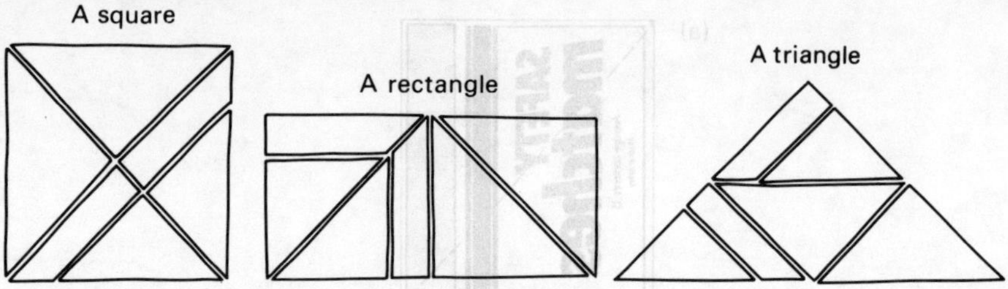

10-5

Make a shape of your own. Draw around it and challenge a friend to make the shape.

For example, David made the shape in figure 10-6 from the six pieces. It is attractive because it has a line of symmetry.

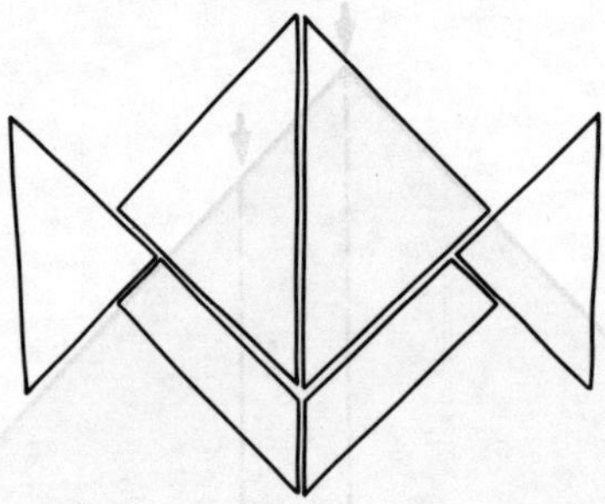

10-6

Children can gain a deeper understanding of area from puzzles like this. Each shape made from the six pieces may look quite different but each has the same area.

Child-to-child activity

The children in your class can make up simple puzzles for their younger brothers and sisters to solve by using just two or three pieces.

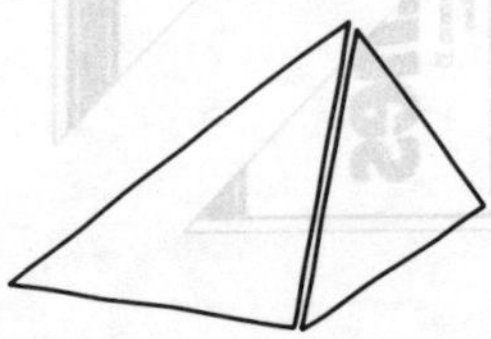

10-7

Example: Use two pieces to make the shape in figure 10-7 or just cut the matchbox into only four pieces and make up puzzles using the four triangles (figure 10-8).

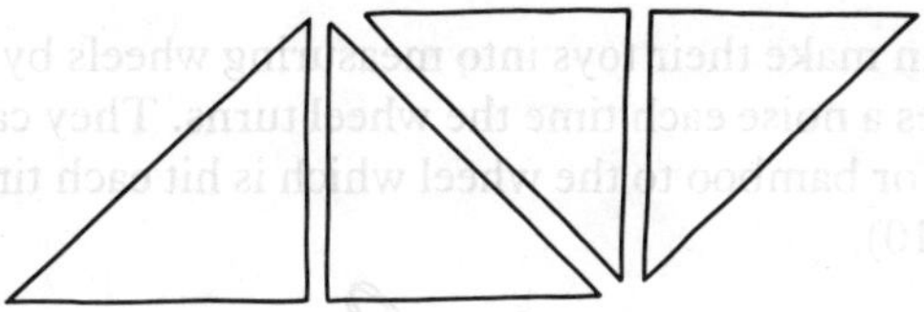

10-8

Here is another very simple way children can make a shape puzzle.

- Stick a picture on to a piece of card.
- Cut into a few pieces.
- Mix up the pieces and see if young children can put the picture back together again.

• Activity 3 Middle

• Measuring distance with tins and wheels

Class activity

Many children play with tins, tyres, hoops or wheels (figure 10-9).

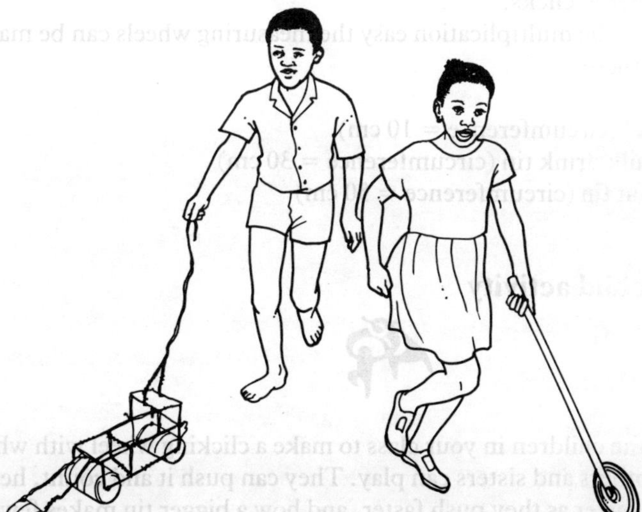

10-9

Here is a way to use this children's game in a mathematical way.

Ask the children to bring to school toys they have made which can be pushed to roll along the ground. The children can measure the circumference of their wheels.

The children can make their toys into measuring wheels by adding a 'clicker' which makes a noise each time the wheel turns. They can do this by adding a piece of tin or bamboo to the wheel which is hit each time the wheel turns (see figure 10-10).

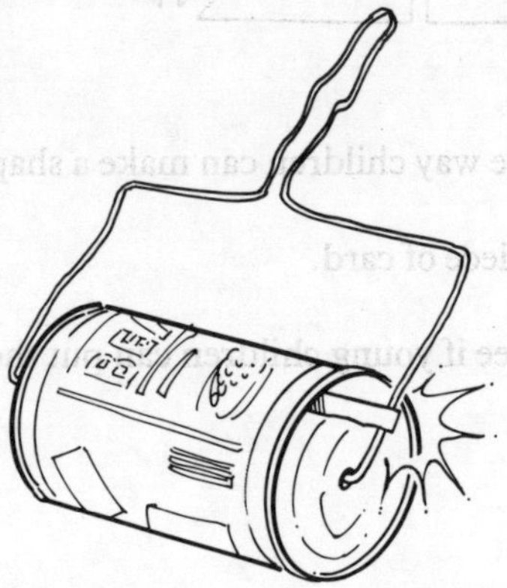

10-10 How to add a 'clicker' to a push-along wheeled toy

The children can now use their toys to measure distances; they can push the toys and count the clicks.

To calculate the distance travelled, the children multiply the circumference by the number of clicks.

To make the multiplication easy the measuring wheels can be made from objects like these:

- cotton reel (circumference = 10 cm)
- malted milk drink tin (circumference = 30 cm)
- cooking fat tin (circumference = 50 cm)

Child-to-child activity

Encourage the children in your class to make a clicking wheel with which younger brothers and sisters can play. They can push it and count, hear how the clicks come faster as they push faster, and how a bigger tin makes fewer clicks than a smaller tin.

• Activity 4 **Middle**

• Capacity of bottles and tins

Class activity

When children learn about capacity they need plenty of practical experience of estimating and measuring.

Ask the children to bring bottles and tins to school. The children can then estimate and measure the capacity of each one. Many bottles have their capacity marked on them. These can be used for measuring other bottles.

For example, some bottles of soft drink hold 300 ml, others hold 200 ml. Using bottles of these two capacities, the children can measure out
(a) 200 ml (b) 300 ml (c) 400 ml (d) 500 ml, and so on . . . .
It is also possible to use them to measure out 100 ml:

- fill the 300 ml bottle with water,
- pour the water into the 200 ml bottle,
- how much is left in the 300 ml bottle?

Child-to-child activity

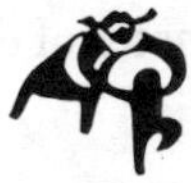

The children can make a collection of containers, plastic bottles, tins, pieces of bamboo, coconut shells. One plastic bottle can be cut to make a funnel.

Playing like this builds up concepts of capacity and volume

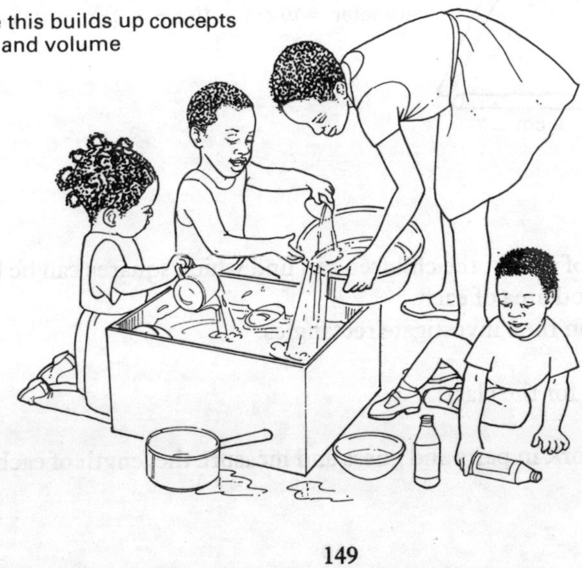

10-11

This collection can be of great educational value to their younger brothers and sisters. Suggest to your class that they help young children to play with the containers, pouring sand and water from one to the other or using them to pretend to mix food (see figure 10-11).

• Activity 5 Middle/upper

• Learning about length and area using sticks

Class activity

Ask each child to bring to school a set of six straight sticks cut so that they have one which is 2 cm long, one 4 cm, 6 cm, 8 cm, 10 cm, and one 12 cm. This is a valuable exercise in careful measurement.

- The children can use the sticks to measure lengths in the classroom using the 10 cm stick as the base.
- The children can investigate how many combinations of the five sticks can be joined to equal the 12 cm stick.
- The children can find how many combinations are possible if *two* sets of sticks are used.
- Using two sets of sticks, the children can investigate how many different triangles are possible and find the perimeter of each, for example, see figure 10-12.

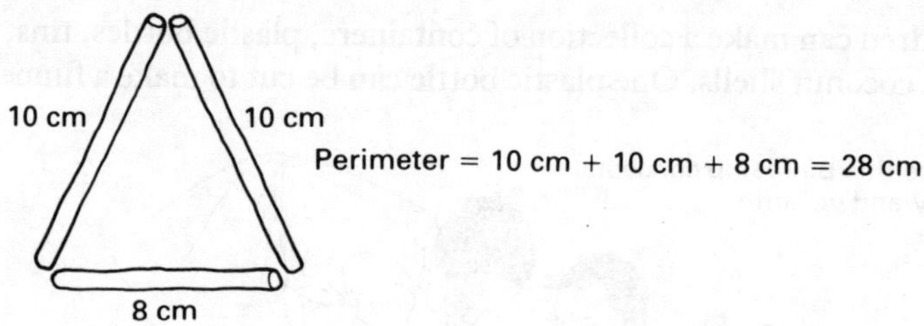

10-12

- Using two sets of sticks, the children can find which squares can be built and the perimeter and area of each.
- The children can then investigate rectangles.

Here is an activity for the class:

- The children work in pairs and guess and measure the length of each other's sticks.

Child-to-child activities

Here are some games that school children can play with younger children using the sticks.

- A guessing game. Hold the sticks in the hand and the children take one each. The longest wins.
- Bury the sticks in the ground so only part is showing. The children try to find the longest one.
- Take one stick and ask the children to find sticks which are shorter.
- Ask the children to arrange the sticks in order of length.
- Hide one stick and see if the children can tell you which is missing.
- Ask the children to find two sticks which join together to make a third.
- Using two sets of sticks, hold one stick up and see if the children can find one equal in length.

• Activity 6 Lower/middle

• Practising addition with dominoes

Class activity

The children can make a set of dominoes from old pieces of card. Measuring and drawing the lines to give 28 rectangular pieces 4 cm by 8 cm is a valuable mathematical exercise. When the pieces are cut out the children can arrange them (see figure 10-13).

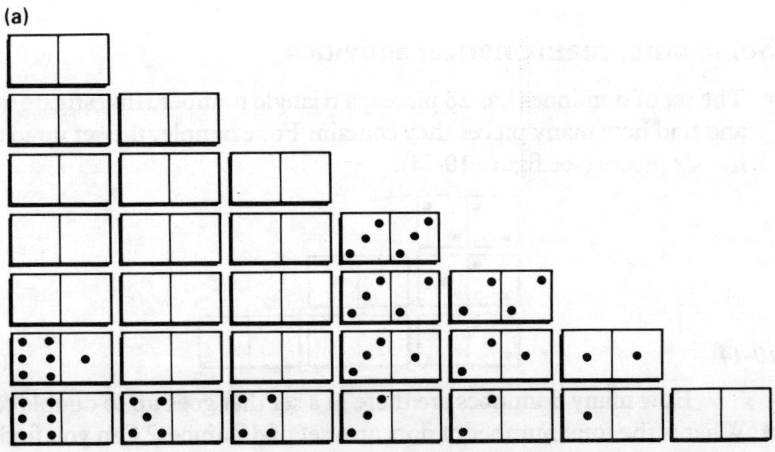

10-13 Start them on the pattern

(b)

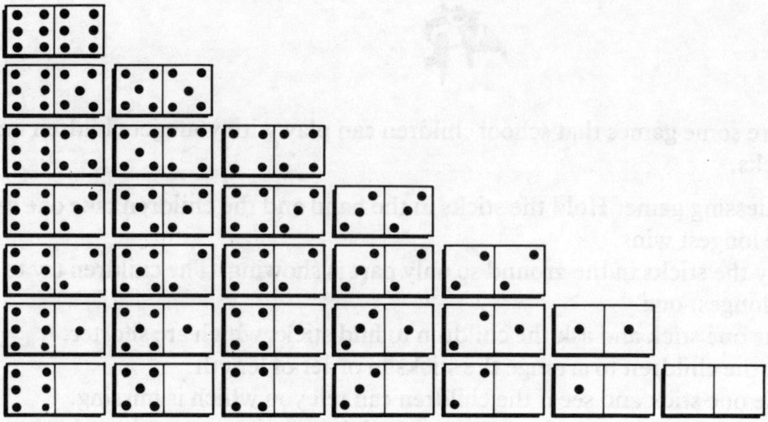

The finished set of dominoes

10-13

Some games to play in class

- Simple matching game: Share out the cards between the players. The player with the double six starts. Each plays in turn, matching to either end of the chain. The first player to use all his/her pieces is the winner.
- Odds and evens: Play in the same way as the simple matching game but now a player scores points depending on the total number of dots when the two ends of the chain are added. If the total is even, the player scores 2 points. If the total is odd, the player scores only 1 point.
- Threes: In this game, players only score points if the total of the two ends is a multiple of 3. The number of points scored is equal to the total divided by 3. Further variations can be played by choosing numbers other than 3 to act as the divisor.

Some other mathematical activities

- The set of dominoes has 28 pieces, a triangle number. Investigate other sets and find how many pieces they contain. For example, the set up to double 2 has six pieces (see figure 10-14).

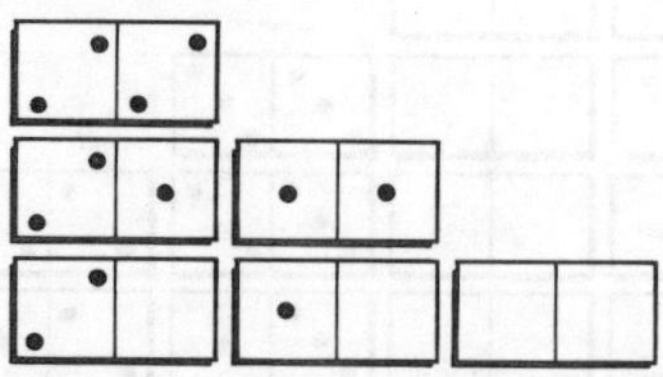

10-14

How many dominoes are there in a set that goes up to double seven?

- What is the total number of dots on a set of dominoes? Can you find a quick way of getting the answer?

Child-to-child activity

- The children can take the dominoes home and teach their younger brothers and sisters to play the simple matching game.

  Playing dominoes at an early age helps children develop pattern recognition and number concepts.
- The children can make a set of picture dominoes in class. Some examples are shown in figure 10-15.

  Playing with this set of dominoes at home will help develop the ability to match shapes.

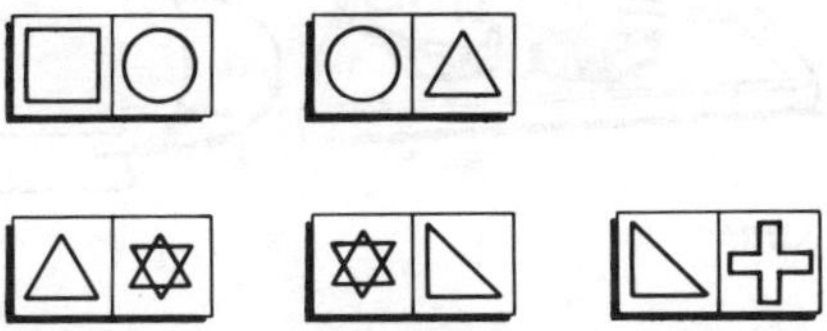

10-15 Some examples of picture dominoes

GAMES FOR OLDER CHILDREN TO TEACH TO YOUNGER CHILDREN

Most of these games school children will enjoy themselves. They are easy to learn and easy to teach and do not need lots of expensive apparatus. Each game, as well as being fun, will teach children about number or shape or pattern.

• Activity 7 — Lower/middle/upper

• Remembering patterns, a memory game

Arrange a set of varied objects in front of young children. Let them look closely and remember each object and its place. Then tell them to close their eyes and while all eyes are closed, take away one object. Hide it behind your back. Then let the children open their eyes. The first child to name the missing object scores a point (figure 10-16).

When you teach this game, first use only a few objects. As the children get better use more and more.

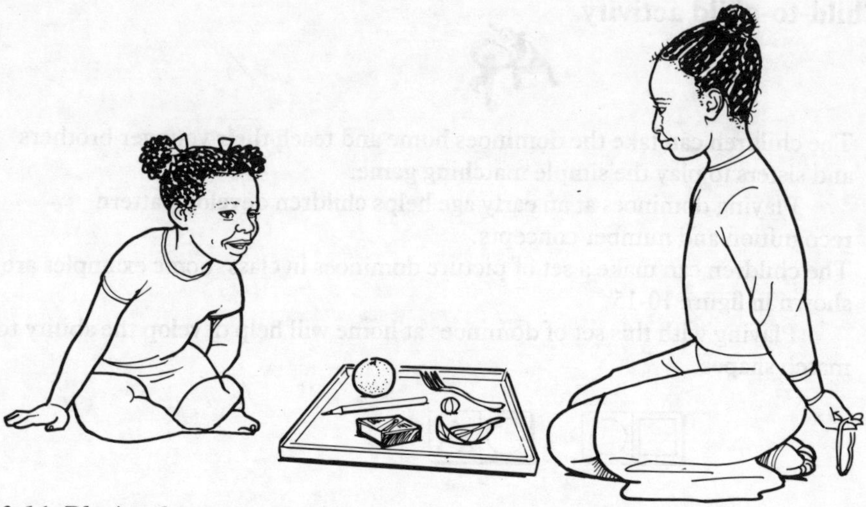

10-16 Playing the memory game

• Activity 8 — Lower/middle/upper

• Looking at shapes, string games

Many children in many different countries teach each other how to make string patterns (see Plate 4). While children play they learn much about shape and pattern.

Find out as many string patterns as possible and teach them to younger children.

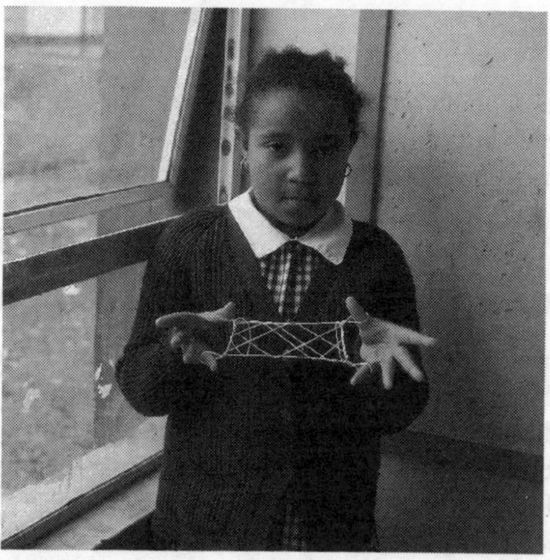

Plate 4 A string pattern

- Activity 9 Lower/middle/upper
- **Making patterns, necklace making**

All over the world people make necklaces from beads and seeds. There is always a pattern and the different beads or seeds follow a definite order. Collect and drill seeds, bottle-tops and small fruits. Then start a pattern for younger children to follow.

- Activity 10 Lower/middle/upper
- **Recognizing shapes, games with leaves**

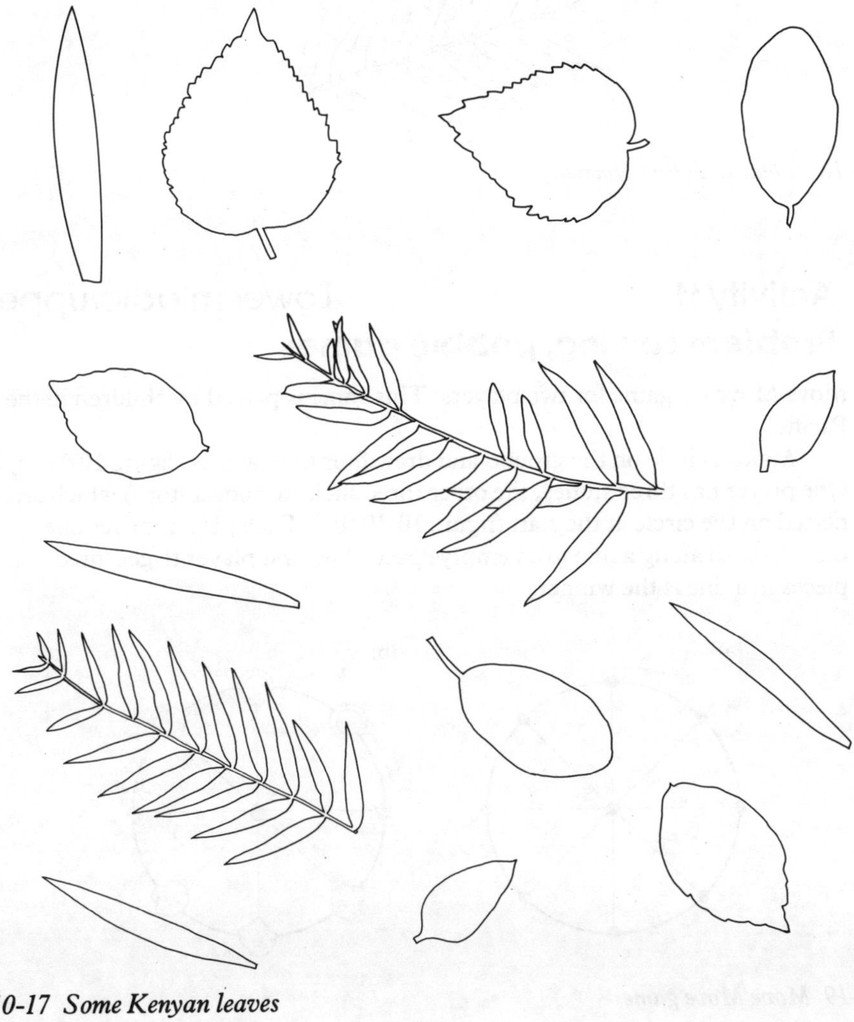

10-17 Some Kenyan leaves

- Collect a variety of leaves, two each from different trees (see figure 10-17). Mix them up and give them to younger children to sort into pairs.
- Gather a set of leaves from the same tree but of different sizes. Ask younger children to arrange them in order of size.
- Tear out pieces from big leaves. Ask younger children to match the torn pieces with the leaf from which it came.
- Find leaves which have line symmetry (see figure 10-18). Pull off some of the leaves from one side. Then get younger children to pull off matching leaves on the other side.

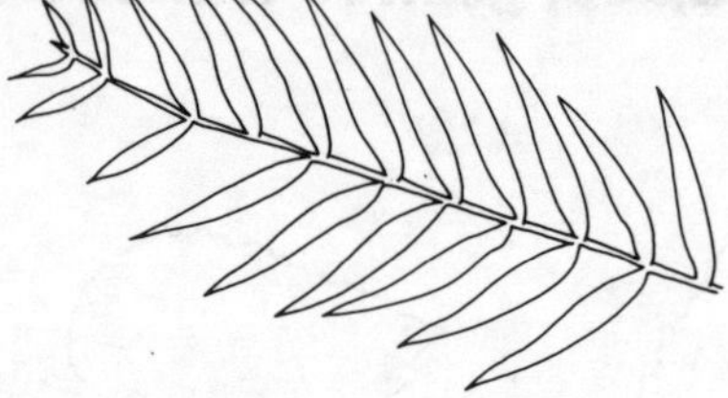

10-18 A leaf with line symmetry

• Activity 11 Lower/middle/upper

• Problem solving, pebble games

- Move Move – a game for two players: This game is played by children in the Pacific.

  Make a circle on the ground and draw four lines across (figure 10-19 (a)). One player has three stones, the other three shells (or bottle-tops) which are placed on the circle at the start (figure 10-19 (b)). Each player moves one piece in turn along a line to an empty space. The first player to get three pieces in a line is the winner.

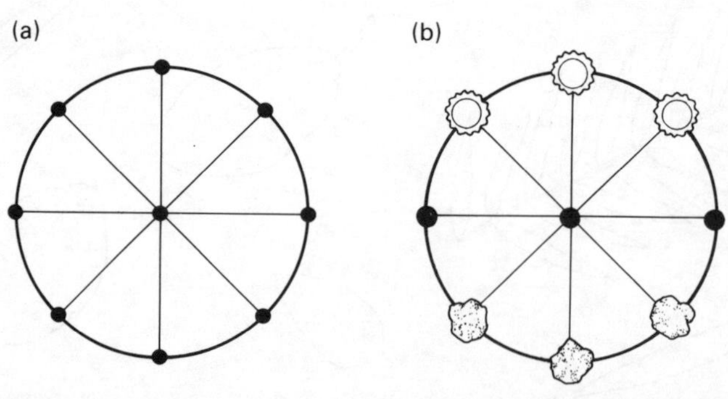

10-19 Move Move game

- Triangle game – a game for two players: Here is a similar game from Africa.

  Draw the board in figure 10-20 (a). Players start by placing their three pieces on the board in turn (figure 10-20 (b)). Then, when all the pieces are on the board, they move a piece in turn to an empty space. The winner is the first player to get three in a line.

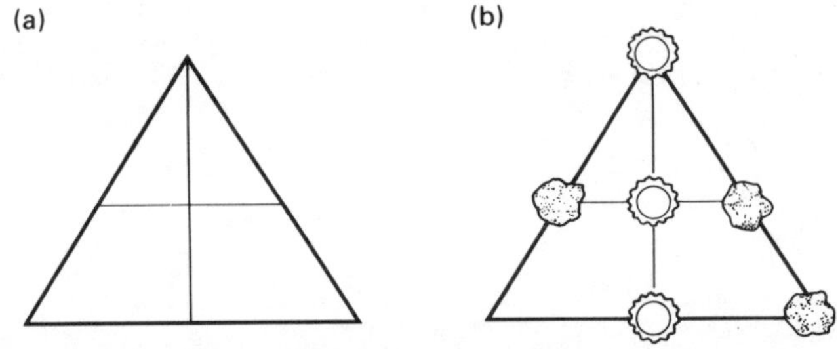

10-20 Triangle game

- Bangura – a game for two to many players: Arrange a lot of stones and one bottle-top in a ring. A number is chosen between 4 and 10. The children take it in turn to count the chosen number around the ring. The stone where each child finishes their count is removed and the next child starts at the next stone in the ring.

  If a child finishes on the bottle-top they are out.
- Mosquito – a game for two players: Put out 12 stones in a line. Each player takes it in turn to take one or two stones. Imagine that under the last stone is a mosquito waiting to bite. The player who takes the last stone loses.

  You can play the game with more stones and allow one, two or three stones to be taken.
- Line game – a game for two or more players: Make up an interesting pattern of pebbles. When the pattern is finished, each child takes a pebble in turn. The first pebble can be taken from anywhere. After this, each pebble taken must be next to the last one taken. The child who takes the last pebble that can be taken is the winner.

  The more interesting the patterns are, the more paths there will be to follow and the more choices to make.
- Stones in hand – a game for two players: Each player has five stones. The players put both hands behind their backs, put some stones in their right hands and place them fist to fist. Each player guesses the total number of stones in the two fists.

  Then the fists are opened and if a player is correct the losing player has to give up one stone.

These are just a few of the many thousands of games played by children throughout the world. Children can be encouraged to teach each other games that they know so that these can be taught to yet more children at home.

Why not ask your class to invent games of their own? You might have a class competition to find the best game they can invent for five-year-olds.

Appendix: How to make a squared blackboard

Having a squared blackboard makes the teaching and learning of many topics much easier. Mark a quarter or a third of your board in squares using either

- a felt pen
- a pencil
- a nail to make a scratch, then rub over the scratch with the board duster and the chalk dust will fill the scratch giving a fine white line which never fades.

The best size of squares to have is 10 cm by 10 cm. To make neat, accurate squares, follow these steps.

Step 1
Make marks 10 cm apart down the board. Make two columns a metre apart. Make the first mark of each column 10 cm from the top of the board.

Step 2
Join the dots horizontally to give parallel lines.

Step 3
Now mark the top and the bottom line at 10 cm intervals. Start 10 cm from the left edge of the board.

Step 4
Join these marks vertically.

It is now easy to draw charts and graphs on the blackboard. It is also much easier for the children to copy your charts and diagrams on to squared paper.

If your supply of squared paper is limited, why not save up exercise books marked in squares and only give out squared paper when you need to use it.

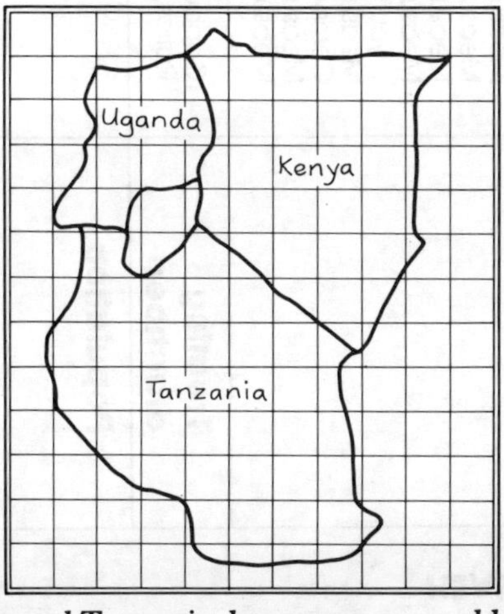

Map of Kenya, Uganda and Tanzania drawn on a squared blackboard

THE HEALTH INTO MATHEMATICS CHART

HEALTH TOPIC	Measurement	Statistics
Body and growth monitoring	Comparing heights p.53 Ordering heights p.54 Measuring height using arbitrary units p.54 Measuring using metric units p.55 Body measurements p.56 Measuring around parts of the body p.57 Measuring grip p.58 Measuring upper arm circumference p.58 Measuring the upper arm circumference of younger children p.60 Measuring heart rate p.67 Comparing heart rate before and after exercise p.68 Measuring breathing rate p.70 Measuring eyesight p.71	The age–height graph p.60 The age–height chart p.61 Measuring the height of younger children p.63 The age–weight chart p.64 Interpreting age–weight charts p.66
Treating diarrhoea	Capacity and volume, measuring with bottle-tops p.126 Ratios, paper cups for sugar–salt solution p.128	A survey of the occurrence of diarrhoea p.125 Statistics on ORT p.129
Population		Position in the family p.11 Life expectancy p.22 Population pictogram p.23 Population statistics p.23 Population pyramids p.28 Counting and comparing using the family tree p.74 Using a pictogram to show birth order p.76 Collecting information, the taller family tree p.76 Tabulating information from a household survey p.77 Combining household surveys p.78 Understanding national data p.78 The range of family size p.90 My family size p.90 Family size and predicting future population p.91 Using a time line to show birth interval p.93

Nutrition and breast feeding		Our favourite growth foods p.13 Our favourite energy foods p.15 Pie charts of how work is shared p.27 Meal survey p.99 Comparing two charts, bottle-top survey p.100 Feeding survey of young children p.102 Statistics of stunted growth p.104 Understanding a chart about breast feeding p.105
Water and sanitation	Capacity and weight of water containers p.133 Measuring distance from a water supply p.134 Statistics on how we use water p.134 Building a school latrine, measuring p.137	Comparing charts of water sources p.132 Toilet survey p.136 Looking at statistics p.138
Infectious diseases and immunization		Last illness p.12 When to take medicines p.19 Illness chart p.20 Infant death rate p.21 Comparing graphs about common diseases p.25 Relating graphs about malaria and rainfall p.25 Class survey p.111 Children survey younger children p.112 Comparing with national data p. 113 Looking at statistics on immunization p.114 Reading information from a table p.115 Illness survey p.118 A running tally of illness p.118
Accidents		Accidents in the household p.16 How do cuts happen? p.17 Road accidents p.17
Health of the growing mind	Measuring distance with tins and wheels p.147 Capacity of bottles and tins p.149 Learning about length and area using sticks p.150 Practising addition with dominoes p.151	
	MATHS TOPIC	

THE HEALTH INTO MATHEMATICS CHART

HEALTH TOPIC	Ratio	Percentage	Problem solving
Body and growth monitoring	Body ratios p.36	From tenths to percentages p.43	Predicting adult height p.63
Treating diarrhoea	Sugar–salt solution p.38 Capacity and volume, measuring with bottle-tops p.126 Sugar–salt solution p.127	Using percentage, death due to diarrhoea p.126 A survey of knowledge about diarrhoea p.130	A cure for diarrhoea, an exercise in ordering p.130
Population	Sex ratios p.31 Age ratios p.34	Birth rate p.46 Infant death rate p.48 Using percentage growth rate p.84	Population statistics p.23 Making predictions using doubling times p.83 Filling squares with dots to show population doubling p.82 A doubling population of folded paper people p.82 To demonstrate the idea of a doubling population p.81 Sharing out land p.86 Calculating land available for farming p.87 Representing population an a map p.87
Nutrition and breast feeding	Understanding ratios, mixing food p.101	Survey of 25 children's favourite fruits p.42 Comparing percentages p.45	Problem solving, buying a balanced meal p.103 Using a weight-for-age table p.106 Using a height-weight table p.107

Water and sanitation	Sanitation ratios p.34		Measuring distance from a water supply p.134 From source to mouth, a flow chart p.135 Using water meters to calculate water use p.139 Costing a water supply p.139
Infectious diseases and immunization	Immunization ratios p.36 Health ratios in the class p.31	Disease survey of 100 children p.40 Class survey p.111 Reading information from a table p.115	Hand touching models the way disease spreads p.119 The touching squares show how disease spreads p.120 The mathematics of the spread of AIDS p.121
Accidents	Health ratios in the class p.31	Accident survey of 20 children p.42 From tenths to percentages p.43	
Health of the growing mind			Kumi puzzles, shapes, symmetry and area p.144 Practising addition with dominoes p.151 Remembering patterns, a memory game p.153 Recognizing shapes, games with leaves p.155 Problem solving, pebble games p.156
	MATHS TOPIC		